To the future generation: Sophia, Lily, and Laura.
May you grow up strong and proud.
And in loving memory of the mothers who raised us:
Patricia Gray and Barbara Phillips.

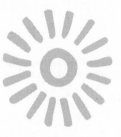

Real Girl Real World
A Guide to Finding Your True Self

by Heather M. Gray & Samantha Phillips

Illustrated by Ellen Forney

Seal Press

Real Girl Real World:
A Guide to Finding Your True Self

Published by
Seal Press
An Imprint of Avalon Publishing Group, Inc.
AVALON
publishing group incorporated
1400 65th Street, Suite 250
Emeryville, CA 94608

Library of Congress Cataloging-in-Publication Data

Gray, Heather M.
  Real girl, real world : tools for finding your true self / by Heather M. Gray and Samantha Phillips.— 2nd ed.
      p. cm.
  Includes bibliographical references.
  ISBN 1-58005-133-2 (pbk.)
    1. Teenage girls—Psychology—Juvenile literature. 2. Self-esteem in adolescence—Juvenile literature. 3. Self-perception in adolescence—Juvenile literature. 4. Sexual ethics—Juvenile literature. 5. Beauty, Personal—Juvenile literature.   6. Feminine beauty (Aesthetics)—Juvenile literature.
  I. Phillips, Samantha. II. Title.

HQ798.G68 2005
305.235'2—dc22
                              2004028528

ISBN 1-58005-133-2

9 8 7 6 5 4 3 2 1

Cover Illustration by Ellen Forney
Cover design by Dayna Navaro
Interior design by Diane Rigoli
Printed in the Canada by Transcontinental
Distributed by Publishers Group West

The authors are not medical doctors. They advise seeking professional medical care for all medical concerns.

Contents

Chapter 2

Body Image–Can't Get No Satisfaction?

Chapter 3

Eating Disorders–When Eating Goes Way Out of Order

Chapter 4

Take a Good Look Down There–Menstruation, Anatomy, Orgasms, and Masturbation

Chapter 5

Coming to Terms with Our Sexuality

Chapter 6

Being in Charge of Our Sexuality

Chapter 7

Feminism—What Is It, and Do We Care?

Conclusion: Be True to Yourself Always 229

Note to the New Edition

While working on this new edition of *Real Girl Real World*, we asked ourselves: What is important to girls now? Are the issues that girls face the same or different nearly a decade later? What can this book give to girls today?

We believe the issues we covered in 1998 are still alive today and that some have been taken by our culture to even greater extremes. While the world faces pressing issues like the ongoing AIDS pandemic and mounting war casualties, the popular media overemphasize such scintillating topics as: celebrity wardrobes, bachelor and bachelorette breakups, who's hot and who's not, lawsuits of the rich and infamous, and the latest impossible diet phenomenon. Among the media frenzy over mean girls, internet hookups, extreme makeovers, young stars' eating disorders and sexual escapades, there's little discussion of the everyday achievements and incredible accomplishments of young women.

This imbalance in the media has troubling consequences. A quick look at recent headlines and studies reveals that young women are struggling more than ever with body image issues: Identification with TV stars and models positively correlates with body dissatisfaction;[1] "Idealized Women in TV Ads Make Girls Feel Bad";[2] "Health Epidemic: Why Are So Many Girls Cutting Themselves?" [3] The sexuality and sexual activity of young girls are also topics of concern; a recent study found that "12–14 year olds appear to be experimenting with a wider range of sexual behaviors at progressively younger ages,"[4] and every year, nearly four million new sexually transmitted infections occur among fifteen- to nineteen-year-olds.[5] Yet the American government insists on giving schools incentives to teach abstinence-only sex education. These "just say no" sex ed classes ignore the fact that more than half of seventeen-year-olds have had intercourse and that all teens, sexually active or not, would like real information, not catchy slogans. The road through girlhood is fraught with land mines. We believe that *Real Girl Real World* gives girls the support and information that is so often missing in our media-saturated, fast-paced lives.

Adolescence is a unique time when we begin figuring out who we are and what is important to us. It is a time for exploring our independence, our voice, and our dreams. It is not a time for being perfect or having it all figured out. Perhaps more than any other time in our lives, as teens we are naturally open, curious, and flexible. And so it is tragic when we soak up messages that, in the interest of selling us something, tell us over and over again that we are not good enough, that we need to morph into a superstar version of ourselves in order to feel successful or content. These self-serving cultural messages are misleading, and can have a very negative effect on our self-confidence and self-image. And it gets especially difficult to ignore these messages when they are slipped in between the glamorous and glossy pages of magazines, sold to us in products, and repeated subtly but steadily through our entertainment channels. If anything, the marketing world has only gotten better at delivering these destructive messages to us in the last eight years.

Real Girl Real World is as relevant today as ever because we still need a book that speaks the truth to girls. This new edition offers girls information and resources on a variety of issues, such as: why the beauty culture is more about consumerism than helping us feel beautiful; ways we can become media savvy; how body dissatisfaction leads to self-destruction and what we can do to build body acceptance; why diets don't work and how to avoid eating-disordered behavior; how to explore our sexuality and stay healthy at the same time; and where to learn about activists who are creating new opportunities for girls and women. This new edition is an upgrade in every way, with more resources, facts, and information to help girls honor their true selves. We hope this book helps to give the world more of what it needs: girls who are growing up strong and proud.

Please check out our new website that offers additional information and resources at www.realgirlrealworld.com.

Samantha Phillips and Heather M. Gray
Miami and New York City
October 2004

Introduction

We decided to write *Real Girl Real World* after wasting so much of our time thinking we'd figure out life if we could just figure out how to look good. *Real Girl Real World* is not about telling you who you should be or what you should look like, or about giving you a glossed-over picture of life. Instead, you'll get real girls' experiences and resources that show you there's no one "right" way to be. *Real Girl Real World* covers issues central to girls' lives, whether we want them to be or not: beauty, body image, sexuality, and feminism. There is also a lot of humor in this book because the media give us laughable and even ridiculous solutions to the problems and issues that girls face. Take a look at this slogan: "Go ahead. Discover who you *really* are. Say hello to Splashin' Lovely Body Sprays." Discover yourself by spritzing your body with perfume? Maybe not. This book encourages you to sift through all the messages you get about being a girl and becoming a woman, to throw out what you don't like, to find out what you do like, and—most importantly— to be happy with who you are.

Teen girls are a hot topic. Studies and books have come out about the downfall of teenage girls. The American Association of University Women surveyed three thousand girls and boys, ages nine to fifteen, and found that girls experience a huge drop in their self-esteem during adolescence, especially when compared to their male peers.[1] A media blitz began in the 1990s, partially ignited with the release of such books as *SchoolGirls*, *Reviving Ophelia*, and *Odd Girl Out*. These books put girls in the limelight, asking why girls are struggling with problems such as academics, body image, and a lack of goals. Suddenly, everyone seemed to be asking, "What's happening to our daughters?"

The results of all those studies were not such a mystery or surprise to us. As girls, we get crazy images of who we are supposed to be: heroines who live happily-ever-after with Prince Charming, models in magazines who are always upbeat, and women who diet to succeed. Parents or friends can be unaware of the pain—both emotional and physical—caused by their suggestion that we need to lose a few pounds. Relationships on TV are about guys chasing beautiful girls (female characters who don't fit the generic beauty mold are side characters without a date). We rarely get straight facts on important issues, such as why diets can be bad for us, or how to avoid STIs and pregnancy. We may be told that we can do anything boys can do, like run for Congress or anchor the evening news, but we also get the message that we'd better look stylish and pretty while doing so. Magazines shout that the key to success is the right combination of cosmetics, cleavage, and the latest fashion accessories. We're told that math class is tough for us and chided for "throwing like a girl." A lot of these messages directly counteract our own instincts—we know deep down inside that we deserve to be strong, feel good, act smart, and have fun.

We would have appreciated an honest look at female teen issues when we were growing up. *Real Girl Real World* raises questions that need to be openly discussed and offers resources that can get you on the path to finding or preserving your true self. In this book, girls address topics that may help you answer the following questions for yourself:

- Why are beauty and a perfect body supposed to be the keys to my happiness?
- How come it's such a big deal when I assert myself?
- What are the complex feelings that accompany an eating disorder?
- Is PMS all in my head?
- What is the first sexual experience really like?
- Why does it seem as if only girls get bad reputations?
- What issues will I face as a lesbian or bisexual girl?
- If I want to have sex, how can I avoid getting pregnant or getting a sexually transmitted infection?
- What exactly does "abstinence" mean, anyway?
- Is oral sex safe?
- How does feminism relate to me?

The following chapters show that we are never alone in our experiences, whether we're worrying about fitting in, suffering from an eating disorder, or wondering about our sexuality. Through a collage of stories, facts and humor, *Real Girl Real World* puts society's messages in perspective and encourages you to express your true self. Each chapter also presents resources such as books, organizations, and websites that offer perspectives other than those of the mainstream media. In these sidebars you'll find alternative information, such as websites at the forefront of the fat liberation movement, tips on how to avoid diets that hurt your health, materials about the latest safer sex methods, and books by hip, young feminists.

We were deeply impressed with the real girls we talked to for this book. Their stories are not dry statistics but rather the thoughts and experiences of real people with attitude, intelligence, and responsibility. We are sure that their voices—and yours—will resonate with one another and be heard by society at large, now and in the future.

Enjoy,
Samantha and Heather, 1998

1

The Beauty Standard
Wasting Our Time on Perfection

Every society has its idea of beauty, and it teaches it to every generation in whatever way necessary.

When you're a baby, people tell you that you are pretty, or they don't. People tell you who else is pretty, like, "Look at that pretty lady!" They are talking to a baby, and it never stops.

—Rebecca, seventeen years old

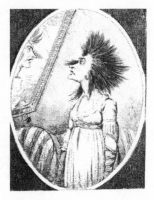

From the moment we're born, girls are greeted with, "Ooh, how pretty, delicate, and lovely." Our brothers, meanwhile, are told, "What a slugger! What a grip—he'll be an athlete!" Goo-goo. From day one we are taken for a ride about prettiness and beauty. So fasten your seatbelts—it's a bumpy trip. Bows are taped to our baby-bald heads. We're given dolls to primp and dress up and frilly party dresses that we can't party in. Even if we are tomboys and never play with dolls or wear dresses, we can't escape the pretty culture. We grow up among pictures of waifish supermodels, fairy tales of beautiful princesses who live happily ever after, buxom blond Barbie dolls with permanently arched "high-heeled" feet, and a constant stream of commentary by the adults around us about what's pretty and what's not.

I'd like to think that beauty is defined as being a good person, but I don't think it works out that way in our society.

Basically, the beauty that everyone thinks they should be is what they see on TV, in movies, and in magazines. Personally, I like people who look a little different.

—Keisha, seventeen years old

> i think pretty is nice
> but i'd rather see something new
> all those plastic people
> got their plastic surgery
> but we got a big big beautiful
> we got it for free
> who you gonna be
> if you can't be yourself
> you can't get it from tv
> you can't force it on anybody else

—Ani DiFranco, "Pick Yer Nose," *Puddle Dive*

The Importance of Beauty: What a Headache

> What else do they want in life but to be as attractive as possible to men? Do not all their trimmings and cosmetics have this end in view? And all their baths, fittings, creams, scents, as well—and all those arts of making up, painting, and fashioning the face, eyes, and skin? Just so. And by what other sponsor are they better recommended to men than by folly?

—Erasmus, 1509

Beauty is made out to be a girl's greatest achievement in life. We are judged more on our looks than on our actions. Sportscasters comment on how pretty or cute female ice skaters and gymnasts are. Can you imagine them complimenting football players on their uniforms or wrestlers on their hairstyles? We get a sinking feeling that it is more important to be beautiful than to be creative, talented, or intelligent. Beauty: the ultimate source of power for women? That stinks. It's fine if I am an accomplished pianist, great writer, adept athlete, or math wiz, but more importantly, *How do I look?* How we look shouldn't matter so much. It *is* possible to throw away the notion that beauty is our most important quality. We can start by reading fashion magazines with a grain of salt and realizing that beauty does not have to be our burden. We can critique what we don't like in the media and choose alternatives to mainstream images. For some cool and different views on the whole beauty scene, check out the sidebar on page 20.

We learn to be beautiful as the way to get a powerful guy.

Men have so many more chances in life if they are not good-looking. It's universal, isn't it? There is a saying for young girls: "Just be beautiful and shut up." People often say, "Oh, the man is rich, that is why he has such a beautiful woman." But sometimes she has everything: the looks, the career, yet she chooses an ugly man, and it's not an issue. Yet if it's the other way around, you think, "That ugly woman must have a lot of money," or "What happened?" In Haiti we would wonder, "Did she do some voodoo to get him?" We are all so conditioned. We learn to be beautiful as the way to get a powerful guy, but who wants someone who's just interested in how we look?

—Marie, eighteen years old

It's like you're not even a real woman if you don't look beautiful.

I think men have more leeway. Even though they are supposed to be built, it is not stressed nearly as much as it is for women. Sure, attractive men get attention, but it isn't like all men have to look attractive to be accepted. But for women, I think it's like you're not even a real woman if you don't look beautiful. Look at Woody Allen. He is a total nerd, but he is sexy. That is great, but it saddens me that it isn't that way for women. You have to live up to so much—it's really frustrating.

—Morgan, seventeen years old

Cover Teasers from Popular Fashion Magazines

"Top 10 Reasons You're Having a Bad Hair Day"

"Flawless Skin Overnight"

"92 Best New Beauty Finds"

"The 50 Best Hair Tips Ever!"

"Makeup's Hot New Colors"

"What's Sexy Now!"

"Get Bulge Free in 28 Days"

"Resize Your Thighs: Moves to Firm Your Most Flab-Prone Body Part"

"Improve Me! How Five Experts Would Make You Beautiful"

Feeling Ugly: Beauty and Self-Esteem

I don't look at faces
I look at my feet
I'm all alone when I walk down the street
I'm in the kitchen 'cause I can't take the heat
I want to live but I stay in my seat
Because I'm ugly with a capital "U"
and I don't need a mirror to see that it's true

—Juliana Hatfield, "Ugly," *Hey Babe*

On a good day, I can see dark brown eyes, long lashes, a sensual mouth, smooth skin, and an endearing nose. On a bad day these are eclipsed and only the bags under my eyes, wrinkles, kinky hair, fat lips, and a pug nose are visible. On a terrible day, there's almost nothing to see at all except a blur of indefensible humanity as I avert my gaze. And on a glorious day, the beautiful eyes behold me, full of love, humor, and intelligence.

—Kathrin Perutz, *Beyond the Looking Glass*

How we feel about ourselves and how we feel about our looks are often tangled together. One day everything is going swell, and we look in the mirror and think, "No problem." Another day nothing is going right, and we look at ourselves and think, "Yuck."

We may put our lives on hold while we chase after a slippery beauty ideal that is not based on who we are: "As soon as I lose these couple pounds, then my life will work out," "Once my acne clears up, I'll have the perfect boyfriend," or "When I get my hair smooth and straight, everything will be great." Rather than striving to fit the beauty images we are presented with, we can choose to appreciate ourselves right now. We can celebrate our own ethnic look, our unique height and shape, and our own real hair color.

I learned you don't have to look at the pictures.

When you look at magazines and you see those models, sometimes you feel bad about yourself. If you're a little bit overweight, you think, "Wow, I'm fat." That's the way I looked at it, but I learned you don't have to look at the pictures. If you

Here She Comes, Miss America

Stories about competitions to find the most beautiful woman have been around for thousands of years. According to the book of Esther, more than two thousand years ago, the king of Persia created a beauty contest to find a queen, and beautiful young virgins from far and wide were paraded in front of him for his approval. The girls had spent a year preparing for the contest—six months softening their skin with oils and six months practicing applying perfumes and cosmetics. Queen Esther gained her crown by winning the contest.

The first Miss America beauty contest was held in Atlantic City in 1921. A group of businessmen thought they could boost tourism past Labor Day by holding a beachfront bathing beauty contest. There were eight contestants, and it was called a "National Beauty Tournament." The winner was Margaret Gorman, a sixteen-year-old blond. Samuel Gompers (president of the American Federation of Labor) said this about the winner: "She represents the type of womanhood America needs. Strong, red-blooded, able to shoulder the responsibilities of homemaking and motherhood. It is on her type that the hope of the country rests." All for a sixteen-year-old who was considered the "prettiest"! The beauty-contest idea took off. By 1954, the Miss America pageant was broadcast live from coast to coast and is now seen around the world. In 2004, a record low 9.8 million people watched the pageant in the United States—about 500,000 fewer than the year before. The ratings have been declining for eight out of the past ten years.[1] (Does the show need a makeover?) Currently, the show awards college scholarships—that's nice, but still hard to reconcile with the mandatory bathing suit competition. Some ask, is scholarly merit based on intellect, or on how we look in a swimsuit?

The Miss America pageant was chosen as the site of one of the first modern-day feminist protests in 1968. The protest was based on the belief that the contest reflected women's role as "passive decorative objects."

don't like yourself, it's okay to try to change it, but you have to realize you can't change much. You have to deal with how you look.

—Tanisha, fourteen years old

I find I'm really not okay if I don't feel pretty.

If I don't feel I look good, then I don't approach people as easily. I've always envied people who could just be themselves no matter how they looked and be out- going all the time. But I find I'm really not okay if I don't feel pretty that day. I shouldn't feel that one day I look good and the next I don't. I'm the same person.

—Valerie, seventeen years old

Fairy Tales: Pretty Little Princesses

In kindergarten, we cuddled up to our teachers at story time and lis- tened to tales of beautiful princesses who lived "happily ever after." We learned that beauty is the key to a happy life. In fairy tales, there are two types of female characters: the evil ones who are ugly, and the good ones who are beautiful. The heroines of these tales—whether Cinderella, Snow White, Sleeping Beauty, or Ariel of *The Little Mermaid*—are the "prettiest in the king- dom" or the "fairest of them all." And they all have long, luxurious hair. (Try to imagine a fairy princess with a nice crew cut!) What does their magnificent beauty get them? Why, Prince Charming himself, and the chance to ride off into the sunset. There is never much action on the heroine's part; in fact, she is often suspended in a kind of limbo, waiting for her prince to rescue her. The moral of the story always seems to be: Be beautiful, and it will all work out. If we were to believe these tales, we should all be sitting in front of the mirror, waiting for our prince to ride in on his white horse.

Luckily, some modern fairy tales give the female heroine more active and diverse roles than the traditionally passive and pretty princess. Let's visit a classic prototype, and then an excerpt from the hip tale *The Paper Bag Princess* by Robert Munsch.

• • •

Once upon a time, there was a princess who was the prettiest creature in the world. Her hair glittered, waved, and rippled nearly to the ground, her dresses were embroidered with diamonds, and everybody who saw her fell in love with

I see that life is not just about, 'If I looked beautiful then I'd be happy.'

My roommate is a model, and she is the embodiment of my concept of beauty. It is hard to deal with her without being jealous or resentful or in awe. A lot of times I feel intimidated by her and don't want to get close to her because she is not an equal, she is this gorgeous untouchable. It's hard for me not to feel less than beautiful around her. At times I can see her as a person—she is a nice person who I get along with and have things in common with. It helps to know she has problems too—she's not entirely confident about what she looks like, she has bad days too. I see that life is not just about, "If I looked beautiful then I'd be happy."

—Kelly, eighteen years old

her. A prince called Charming came to the kingdom and decided he must have her hand. He was very brave and strong. One day, Charming and Princess Lovely went for a walk in the woods. A giant tried to attack them, so Charming pulled out his shining sword while Lovely trembled in fear. With one fell swoop, Charming cut the giant's head off and saved the day. Upon their return to the kingdom, the two got married and lived happily ever after.

. . .

[Elizabeth] was going to marry a prince named Ronald.

Unfortunately, a dragon smashed her castle, burned all her clothes with his fiery breath, and carried off Prince Ronald.

Elizabeth decided to chase the dragon and get Ronald back.

She looked everywhere for something to wear, but the only thing that she could find that was not burnt was a paper bag. So she put on the paper bag and followed the dragon. . . .

[With her own cunning, Elizabeth tired out the dragon, and he fell sound asleep.]

Elizabeth walked right over the dragon and opened the door to the cave.

There was Prince Ronald. He looked at her and said, "Elizabeth, you are a mess! You smell like ashes, your hair is all tangled, and you are wearing a dirty old paper bag. Come back when you are dressed like a real princess."

"Ronald," said Elizabeth, "your clothes are really pretty and your hair is very neat. You look like a real prince, but you are a bum."

They didn't get married after all.

Sometimes I'll wish my eyes were bigger, and my nose was narrower, and that I just looked more white in general.

But now I try not to compare myself to non-Asians; I just compare myself to other Asians. Ideally, I wouldn't compare on looks at all, but just on personality.

—Yun, seventeen years old

I realized that there are also some advantages to not being that beautiful.

When I was fifteen, almost all the girls in my grade were very beautiful. All the boys in high school wanted to get to know them. I was not considered beautiful because I didn't dress up, and I have a big face and my body is round. I didn't feel like an attractive girl who people would like. This feeling of insecurity took a huge effort to surpass. It was really a crisis, and I had to find some confidence. One of the things I gained from this experience is I am not so fragile. I don't need to feel beautiful.

When two friends came to visit me, everyone said they were such pretty girls. But I realized that there are also some advantages to not being that beautiful. One of the girls, who is dating this popular guy, told me that she feels lonely. She thinks it might be because she has had too much success with men. She says she feels more sad than happy when everyone likes her because she doesn't like herself. What I like the most in my relationships with people is not whether they consider me beautiful or ugly but that they like me as a person.

—Anya, seventeen years old

Models of Beauty: A Split Second Captured on Film

She has a perfect body.

I admire the model Nikki Taylor because she's very pretty; she has a perfect body. She has really nice hair, and I like her beauty. Nope, there's no one else I admire.

—Nina, fourteen years old

When more than five hundred girls in _____ twelve were asked which women they admired most, th_____ ____ ove writers, actresses, singers, politicians, and ___ ____ ____ lights our flimsy perceptions of cultural su_____ ____ ____ecting the women around us for their intell_____ ____ ____ore often look up to the models we see in fa____ ____ ____, because we are admiring a moment in time, a split ____ ____ ___.

Hooray! I hear you admiring all kinds of women for all kinds of reasons!

Our readers will not embrace an overweight model with zits. We
don't give them exactly who they are. [The readers] are aspiring
to something.

–Sally Lee, former editor at YM

What a joke. It's insulting to be handed such a narrow definition of beauty to
"aspire to," especially since we live in a world full of diversity. It would be a different
story if magazines showed us hundreds of looks and body types, of which the white,
skinny, tall type were just one. Then everything would be groovy. It's a drag that
those glamorous, touched-up faces and bodies are nearly the only images of beauty
presented to us. We are fooled into thinking that to be beautiful, we have to look like
fashion models.

Some modeling agents report receiving four hundred phone calls a day and five
thousand pieces of mail a week from girls wanting to be the next Naomi Campbell
or Claudia Schiffer.[2] These hopefuls are in for a rude shock, however, because statistically, it would be easier to be elected to the United States Congress than to become
a supermodel! If we're not white, the
odds are even worse: Though about
one out of four Americans is non-
white, only a small handful of supermodels are women of color. Another
bitter truth is that the average female
model is five feet, nine and a half
inches tall and weighs 110 pounds,
whereas the average American
woman is five feet, four inches tall
and weighs 142 pounds.[3] The beauty
ideal we are taught to aspire to is
simply impossible for most women to
achieve.

Train to Be a Model

Train to be a model . . . or just
look like one. Gain popularity!
Confidence! Poise!

–Barbizon

Model Facts:
There are more than 3 billion
women in the world and less than
ten of them are considered to be
supermodels of the moment.[1]

Only 5 percent of the female
population is genetically predis-
posed to look like today's fashion
models. This means it is an impossible goal for 95 percent of women.[2]

cindy, oh cindy
you've sold your soul
to be that girl next door
that sexy unattainable thing.
squashing more young female hearts
than you can imagine

poet laureates?
quantum physicists?
daring philosophers?
no. we need to be pretty.
then things are cool.
then old farts will ogle us,
ridiculous studs will prey on us.

be aloof. be mysterious.
smile, always smile.
don't reveal too much.
that's the ticket.
give us some more makeup tips, cin.
wink, wink. girlfriend.

yeah, well this chick has always
wanted more.
to scale the mountains,
live through the depths,
speak with god,
touch life . . .

—Heather M. Gray

I want to see magazines that reflect what I see on the street and at my school.

Magazines think that the public doesn't want to see real people. The typical teen magazines only show their definition of beautiful people. I hate how they exclude any overweight or "too ethnic-looking" people. They might be in the article sections, but they are never in the fashion or beauty sections. Magazines should

include models who are more realistic in their body type and in their race. I want to
see magazines that reflect what I see on the street and at my school.

—Yvonne, fourteen years old

The things that aren't perfect give you personality.

*When I saw models in magazines, I used to think, "Oh, they're perfect! I'd like
to be perfect too." Now I understand that I wouldn't like to be perfect. Why? Because
the things that aren't perfect give you personality. I don't think the portrayal of models is realistic. Women aren't so perfect—it's not natural.*

—Angela, sixteen years old

It kills me to hear a girl say, "I look so ugly."

*I'm very satisfied with my looks; sometimes I think I'm vain. When I read
magazines and they say how to put makeup on to accentuate your cheekbones or*

Picture Perfect: More Than Meets the Eye

What can be changed in retouching photographs? "You can shrink heads, change eye color, skin color, add people, add clothes—any special effect that you can do in the movies you can do with stills. It's just a question of how much money the art director or photographer wants to spend," says David Terban, a digital artist and an expert in creating those images we all see as we turn the pages of any fashion or beauty magazine. According to Terban, readers should look at all these glamorous pics in good fun because "no one really looks that way. The only crazy part is a lot of the models really are that skinny."

The fashion industry likes to argue that fashion magazines are like the movies: one big fantasy with exotic locations that allow the photographer to be an artist and create an ideal look—something to strive for. But isn't it irresponsible to create standards that are essentially unattainable, except through the magic of film and computers?

So next time you check out the cover of a women's magazine and the model's skin is a bit too perfect, even for a fashion model, remember—it just ain't real! Take comfort in this, and love your own *natural* look. Also, check out the sidebar on pages 30–31 for magazines and other resources that present alternatives to the unattainable look.

Model Talk

The media make it seem as if models never have a bad day—all those glamorous locations, fancy clothes, and oh-so-cool expressions. In reality, modeling can be a tiring, pressured, and competitive experience. Two models talk about what life is like in the fast lane:

You get tired of people critiquing you all the time.

Modeling is a constant reassurance that someone thinks you look good, and most people don't get that kind of approval. Every day it's like, "Well, you're pretty enough to be in this magazine." It's kind of glamorous. You get to wear cute clothes and dress up. But at the same time, you're constantly getting rejected and being told what's wrong with you: "You're too thin," "You should stay the way you are," "Your nose is too big," "You have a nice ethnic look," "Your eyes are too close together," "Your eyes are too far apart." Everything. Sometimes you get really paranoid and think they're right. And you get tired of people critiquing you all the time. I want to shout, "Enough already. I'm sick of being torn apart." But you just have to step away from it and think, "Wait a second, it doesn't really matter." In the end, you have to weigh it out because some people will always think you look good and some people won't.

—Shannon, seventeen years old

brighten your eyes, do this, do that, that is trying to make me feel like my cheekbones or my eyes aren't good enough. And I'm already happy with them. I'm not gorgeous, and I have bad hair days, bad skin days, bad everything days. But I'd be a fool to say I'm ugly, and it kills me to hear a girl say "I look so ugly" because they don't. I don't think anyone looks really ugly.

—Jasmine, fourteen years old

I no longer had one idea of beauty, but lots of ideas of beauty.

In junior high, I was into magazines and thought ideal beauty was tall, voluptuous, long hair, and white skin. I was wanting something that I could never be

They don't realize that all the pictures they see are retouched.

*The typical fashion magazines—*Vogue, Glamour, Seventeen, Elle—*are not realistic. The readers don't realize that all the pictures they see are retouched! That means if the model has a wrinkle, they smooth the wrinkle out, or if her eyes are red, they make them white. They can change your body, too, like if there is a bulge of fat under your behind, they can just touch it up on the picture. The retouching and the light have so much to do with the outcome. I mean, these models are sixteen and they never have pimples? Come on, that's too strange. The girls are so skinny they have to twist and pin clothes behind their backs. It is dangerous because women who don't look like that think, "Oh, I have to look like that." They put so much makeup on us. The first thing everyone does after a photo shoot is take it off; you would never recognize us!*

If I could give advice to a girl just starting out in modeling, I would say, you can't trust too many people. Everyone wants something from you, especially if you are young. You also have to travel a lot, and it's so easy to say, "I love to travel," but it's not so easy when you have to leave your family and friends and go to a country where you don't know anyone or speak the language. It sounds fun, but it's not easy.

—Vicki, eighteen years old

because I'm not tall, I'm not voluptuous, and I'm not white. Watching TV also showed me that men want tall and voluptuous women. Then in high school it changed, and I thought women who looked more like me were beautiful: shorter and with dark hair. I no longer had one idea of beauty, but lots of ideas of beauty. Before I thought because I didn't look like the beauty standard, it meant that I wasn't beautiful. I realized that wasn't true and that I didn't have to fit a stereotypical beauty standard. Lots of people can be beautiful. I think the most attractive people have odd facial features, or are ugly and carry it off really well. Those are the most interesting and attractive people to me.

—Aiko, seventeen years old

Magazines are so glamorous—I see it as fun.

I'm obsessed with fashion magazines, but it's more for the clothes than the models. Magazines are so glamorous—I see it as fun, someone else may see it as intimidating. I think it is enjoyable to pick up a magazine and see the newest lines. As opposed to, "Look how beautiful she is, I just have to look like that," I cut pictures out for the clothes or photography. I think the dresses are beautiful even though I could never wear them. Half the outfits they show on runways are not what they really have in the stores; it's to get you excited about the line.

—Soy, seventeen years old

Pretty Girl

I'm beautiful, I'm gorgeous
Don't try to tell me I'm not
I'm sassy, I'm smart
Don't try to make me change this
I've got class, I've got style
Don't try to make me deny this
Don't try to fix me—I'm not broken
Your pages dictate to me how I should look
How I should act, what I should wear
Your ads tell me what I should
Spend my money on to be better
Your photo shoots show me a glimpse
Of that perfection that I will never have
Well, I want to tell you something—so listen up
I don't want that perfection—I've got my own, thanks
And those rules and tips—I've got a brain
I don't want this "charity," these ideas
Because I love myself
I love my mind, I love my body
Don't try to change me, don't try to turn myself against myself.
Because I'll fight back. Hey Nikki, Cindy, Naomi!
Take a look over here. Here's a real
Pretty girl

—Lila, fourteen years old

Barbie: The Plastic Queen of Beauty

Even our *toys* are focused on idealized beauty. Mattel's Barbie, one of the most popular toys of all time, was introduced at the 1959 New York Toy Fair as "Barbie: a shapely teen-age fashion model. She's grown up!" She was a far cry from the cute, pudgy baby dolls girls usually played with—for starters, she had breasts. Now girls had a hand-held version of the unattainable beauty ideal, complete with matching shoes and accessories.

Every second, three Barbie dolls are sold somewhere in the world. Placed head to toe, all the Barbie dolls and her cohorts sold since 1959 would circle the earth more than seven times![4] Through the years, the Barbie population has changed to adapt to the times. In addition to theme dolls such as Circus Star Barbie, Shopping

Barbie Tales

- The first talking Barbie doll—"Teen Talk Barbie," introduced in 1992—created controversy because one of her sentences was, "Math class is tough."

- The Barbie Liberation Organization, a group of concerned parents, feminists, and other activists, launched an effort to free Barbie from her traditional gender shackles. In 1989, they switched the voice boxes of three hundred talking Barbies and talking G.I. Joes, so that Joe asked, "Want to go shopping?" while Barbie warned, "Dead men tell no lies."[1]

- In 1991, the High Self-Esteem Toys Corporation came out with a "Happy to Be Me" doll that was designed to reflect a more realistic female body type than Barbie. The doll, which had a wider waist, larger feet, and shorter legs, never became popular.[2]

- In 2004, Mattel launched a Barbie line of clothes, accessories, and perfume for adult women: "Barbie is about to break out of her curvaceous plastic mold and turn into a living, breathing person," CNN/*Money* reported. Let's see who will actually wear a Barbie-inspired cocktail dress or shoes in public. A separate clothing collection is being released for young girls.[3]

- Women have a 1 in 100,000 chance of looking like Barbie, while men have a 1 in 50 chance of looking like Ken.[4]

Fun Barbie, and Evening Extravaganza Barbie, Mattel has offered career-oriented Barbies (Day-to-Night Barbie and Army Barbie) and non-white Barbies (Native American Barbie, Korean Barbie, Black Barbie, and Hispanic Barbie). There's even a wheelchair Barbie, an admirable addition, except that when she was first available, she and her chair could not fit in the door to the Barbie Dreamhouse. (Sorry, "imperfect" Barbie—*you* have to stay outside!) One thing has remained true about Barbie: her *amazing* proportions. If she were a full-sized woman, she would have a forty-two-inch bust, an eighteen-inch waist, and thirty-three-inch hips! The average *real* woman is roughly thirty-five (bust), twenty-six (waist), thirty-seven and a half (hips). Barbie, it's time to eat some donuts.

Girls have long admired Barbie's appearance and neat outfits, but boys don't seem to like Barbie's counterpart, Ken. They dig action figures, like G.I. Joe, over the leisurely Ken (who lacks a superhero charisma). Girls, you've probably noticed, are not traditionally given action figures but rather *dolls* with an emphasis on appearance. Now a new generation of girls is learning the plastic beauty ideal through the popular doll Bratz. The Bratz, introduced in 2001, have big heads, skinny bodies, and "a passion for fashion." The message of Bratz is very similar to Barbie's: "Take care, stay stylin', and above all else, be BEAUTIFUL!!"[5]

Who would admire a Barbie doll? She is just skinny and blond with big breasts.

—Kimra, thirteen years old

This is my take on Barbie: She's not so bad, she has a cool pink car, a dream house, and Ken tags along on the side.

They have ethnic Barbies now, which is cool. And there are career Barbies. There is room for improvement, though, like they still need to make a plump Barbie.

—Natalie, seventeen years old

Fashion Trends: They Used to Wear *What*?

If you want a girl to grow up gentle and womanly in her ways
and her feelings, lace her tight.

—One man's testimonial to the corset in the late Victorian press

Women's clothing is about much more than function and practicality—it's about the image that we're supposed to project. Last season, for example, fashion magazines stressed being feminine again, telling us, "Dress like a girl!" and "Curves are back!" But the silly thing about trying to look like the latest *Vogue* cover girl or MTV's newest soul queen is that the ideal image changes like the wind.

Fashion trends mirror what's going on around us—whether it's the end of a world war in the 1940s or a boom of women entering executive positions in the 1980s. The following is a look at beauty and fashion trends throughout the twentieth and into the twenty-first century. (Much of this overview is described in *The Changing Face of Beauty* by Sharon Romm.) Each trend has had a "personality" for women to adopt along with the clothing. Watching old movies or period pieces, we might think, "How could women have worn that?" about styles that seem outrageous and impractical. Fifty years from now, women may be saying the same thing about our current beauty and fashion ideals.

Late 1800s–Early 1900s: Corsets Create the "Perfect" Figure

After the conservative Victorian era ended, sexuality became an important part of the beauty standard. Women were supposed to focus on improving their appearance instead of their "far less useful intellect." The ideal figure had large breasts, a small waist, and slim hips. To achieve the impossible figure of this period, women wore corsets and laced them so tightly that some fainted or had to see their doctors for crushed organs. People admired the beauty of older women, and a "willowy seventeen-year-old would have to wait her turn for the limelight."

The Gibson Girl, a popular character illustrated by Charles Dana Gibson, represented this era's standard of beauty. She was dark haired, small waisted, and "athletic but not manly." Her personality was modest and standoffish. The identity of the model for the Gibson Girl was kept a secret, and some wondered if she existed or not. The Gibson Girl was the last time that a beauty ideal was created by a single artist rather than through multiple media images.

1914–1918, World War I: Back to Natural Forms

During this period, women went to work for the war effort. Naturalness became an asset, and the ideal was "simple and sleek." Women's bodies were released from their corsets and allowed to relax into their natural form.

1920s: Short Skirts All the Rage by Mid-Decade

World War I was over, and new technology allowed for more leisure time. Women finally gained the right to vote. The flapper represented the "easy life" and the greater independence of women in the 1920s, and became the new standard of beauty. She shed her layers of petticoats and for the first time wore shorter skirts that allowed easier mobility and showed off her legs. Prior to this time, a woman needed floor-length skirts, as showing her legs was "immodest, ungodly, and sinful."[6] The flapper's rebellious beauty style, including her newly bobbed hair, paralleled the women's movement, changing the established order. Cinema became a force for the first time, with wide-eyed actresses such as Mary Pickford and Clara Bow stepping into the limelight.

1930s: Women Welcome Pants

Fashion magazines began setting and creating the rules for beauty and fashion. The photographic model replaced the high-society woman as the standard for beauty. Good health and a more athletic build were part of being beautiful. For the first time, it became acceptable for women to wear trousers. Wearing men's clothing was fashionable as long as women kept feminine accessories, such as long hair, jewelry, and high heels. Greta Garbo, with her perfect skin and mysterious image, embodied the ideal that women were striving for.

1939–1945, World War II: The Pin-Up Girl Era

The American ideal of beauty was robust good health and "scrubbed, smiling faces." The pin-up became popular among American soldiers. Rita Hayworth, with her long legs, ample buttocks and breasts, and cute nose, epitomized the pin-up girl.

1950s: Hello, Marilyn

Two types of beauty were in the limelight during this decade. The first was an extremely voluptuous woman with a rougher quality than had been seen before. Movie actresses who represented this version of beauty were Ava Gardner and Jane Russell. The second type was a more childlike and passive woman. After the war, women were supposed to resume their roles as housewives, and a woman's greatest success was thought to be a happy marriage and home life. Fashion ideals returned to small waists and full skirts. Girdles acted as modern corsets and were used to achieve the "perfect" figure. Movie actresses who represented this second type were Sandra Dee and Debbie Reynolds, women who "hid their sexuality under ponytails and bobby socks." Marilyn Monroe, the most famous actress from this decade, managed to embrace both categories of beauty by combining a childlike persona with sexiness.

1960s: Thin Is In (Thanks, Twiggy . . .)

Youth reigned and the hippie aesthetic was in. Models bragged about working-class backgrounds, and everyone could be found in blue jeans. Some women spent hours in front of mirrors trying to achieve the "natural" flower child look. Ninety-two-pound fashion model Twiggy, with her long legs, thin waist, and nonexistent hips and breasts, was idealized as the perfect beauty. Women became obsessed with being thin. As the civil rights movement unfolded, black models broke into the all-white confines of the high-fashion world. Motown Records also introduced such black beauties as Diana Ross and Aretha Franklin.

1970s: Feathered Hair, Lip Gloss, and *Charlie's Angels*

Athletic women who were "wholesome yet erotic" became the ideal. Farrah Fawcett, Diana Ross (showing her staying power through the decades), and Cheryl Tiegs were examples of this decade's beauty goddesses. The interesting and unusual were sometimes in style. For example, Lauren Hutton's gapped teeth and Brooke Shields's shaggy eyebrows were part of their popularity. In the late seventies, we saw the beginning of the "how to dress for success" campaigns.

1980s: Yuppies and Frou-Frou Dresses

The sale of women's suits soared between 1980 and 1987. Then suddenly, in 1987, Christian Lacroix introduced twenty-pound dresses of taffeta and hoops for "women who like to dress up like little girls. But sales were disappointing. It seemed as though the advances women had made in the business world were in direct proportion to the backward leaps of the fashion world. Some other looks seen in women's closets during this decade were athletic/spandex, androgynous, gothic, *Flashdance*-inspired, and punk.

1990s: Retro and Grunge

The nineties saw the waif, grunge, and retro-sixties looks come and go. Other retro hits, such as crimped hair, blue eye shadow, bellbottoms, and platform shoes were deemed "back." Body piercings (nose, tongue, and belly button studs joined the jewelry box) and tattoos were hot.

2000s: Sexy

Tiny tanks, skinny jeans, and belly baring are in. Pants and skirts that reveal underwear make G-strings and boxers part of the visible wardrobe. Flaunting sexuality with near nudity, designer labels, and low slung jeans with very expensive and very high heels are among the trends. As always, it's hard to keep up with the latest styles because they change seasonally. Within these trends, we continue to be given advice from fashion magazines: "How to look professional yet sexy," "How to dress to seduce but not look like a tramp," and let's not forget, "How to find a bathing suit that transforms your so-so bod into a '10.'"

The Fashion Folly / The Bull about Beauty

It's easy to feel that looking good is our primary goal in life. Check out these books, which take on the media and put the beauty standard in its place:

Appearance Obsession: Learning to Love the Way You Look by Joni E. Johnston, Deerfield Beach, FL: Health Communications, 1994.

The Beauty Myth: How Images of Beauty Are Used Against Women by Naomi Wolf, New York: Perennial, 2002.

Cosmetics, Fashions, and the Exploitation of Women by Joseph Hansen and Evelyn Reed, New York: Pathfinder Press, 1986.

Hope in a Jar: The Making of America's Beauty Culture by Kathy Peiss, New York: Metropolitan Books, 1998.

The Power of Beauty: Men, Women, and Sex Appeal Since Feminism by Nancy Friday, New York: HarperCollins, 1997.

Real Gorgeous: The Truth About Body and Beauty by Kaz Cooke, New York: W. W. Norton, 1996.

Where the Girls Are: Growing Up Female with the Mass Media by Susan J. Douglas, New York: Times Books, 1994.

Transforming Our Looks: The Big Makeover

In the factory we make cosmetics. In the store we sell hope.

—Charles Revson, founder of Revlon cosmetics

She wants me to go to the mall
SHE wants ME
To put the pretty, pretty lipstick on
She wants me to be like her
She wants me to be like her

I want to kill her
But I'm afraid it might kill me

—Bikini Kill, "Alien She," *Pussy Whipped*

Fashion magazines and advertisements tell us that with the right amount of mascara, the right shade of lipstick, and the right waft of perfume, we'll be happy and fulfilled—just like the models in the pictures. Many, if not most, beauty products offer quick solutions that will "transform" our lives. We imagine, "If I just use this tangerine peel mask for ten minutes once a week, I can get the radiating skin of that model. Then I can have a cute boyfriend like she has in the picture, and have a truly happy life." All from a facial mask—sure!

I almost always wear something or I feel all sickly looking.

Even if I'm alone watching TV, sometimes I'm in the mood to put makeup on. And going out, it's fun to wear makeup, even if it's just lipstick.

—Libbie, seventeen years old

When I wear makeup, I always worry about it.

I wonder, "Do I have lipstick on my teeth? Is my mascara running?" I don't feel like my real self. I don't wear makeup very often. I usually wear it when I'm trying to look more dressed up.

—Jade, sixteen years old

No makeup for me, thanks.

I really don't feel like myself when I even wear just lipstick or blush. And as for foundation, it feels like I'm burying my skin and clogging my pores with gunk.

—Donna, fifteen years old

Beauty products and makeup tips abound in fashion magazines. Occasionally we will find a "Be Happy with Who You Are" article, advocating that we accept our looks and feel confident. But within a page or two, there will be a full description of "Your Best Look—What Works and What Doesn't," an ad for so-and-so's "One-Stop Beauty Solutions," or an article on "Hair Crimes: Don't Get Caught." Beauty products are only a problem when we think we'll change who we are by using them. The truth is, changing our looks rarely changes our problems.

I wouldn't leave the house to go to the store without makeup on.

I was in seventh grade when I first started wearing makeup. I wore a little bit of powder, mascara, and lip gloss. The next year I started wearing full makeup, and I put it on heavy: foundation, eyebrows, eye shadow, eyeliner, mascara, lipstick, blush, everything. I spent hours on my face. In school, every forty-five minutes I would have to touch up my makeup in class. I would pull out my stuff and put it on my desk in the middle of class while the teacher was lecturing. It was like I was hiding behind a mask. I still put on way too much. I wish that I didn't have to. I feel like I have to because I don't want to have any imperfections. I have to be flawless. To this day, I can take between one and two hours putting on makeup each morning. I definitely spend a decent amount of money on makeup.

I decided I wanted to wear makeup not because of my friends but from looking in fashion magazines and television. When I was younger, I wouldn't leave the house to go to the store without makeup on. Never. No one could ever see me without makeup. I could barely let my mother see me without makeup on, that's how bad it was. Now I can go to the store, but I can't go to a party or a club without it on. I would feel naked and ugly. I wear makeup out of insecurity. People tell me, "You look better without all that makeup on," but I don't believe them and I don't care, because I feel comfortable.

—Kyla, sixteen years old

I did try wearing makeup, but my boyfriend said it looked like I had war paint on.

He has a point—putting on lots of makeup can be like going out for the hunt, chasing down a mate, or wearing a mask. I'm just not comfortable with that.

—Sylvia, seventeen years old

Buns, Beehives, Dreads, or Crews: There's So Much to "Do"

As with clothing, we can become a slave to our hair when we feel like we have to keep up with the latest hairstyles. There were the perms of the '50s, the fabulous 'fros of the '60s, the feathering of the '70s, the Lady Di cuts of the '80s, the "Rachels" (Jennifer Aniston's shaggy cut on *Friends*) of the '90s, and the long, smooth, parted-in-the-middle look in the early 2000s. For the most part, the ideal for hair has been based on straight, silky hair, leading to torturous straightening treatments for many

Hair Appeal: Ideas the Industry Is Selling Us

Not All Updos Are Created Equal:
It takes just a few sexy curls to transform a librarian-like bun into this luscious look. If you don't got 'em, buy 'em: Check out your local wig store.

—*Seventeen*, May 1995

Fall in Love:
Discover the Clairol reds collection, inspired by the romance, the fashion, the free spirit of fall. Romantic reds (and curls) are the rage this season.

—Clairol

Reveal Yourself:
Your rich, sultry, gorgeous brunette self.

—John Frieda

Blond Ambition...
Forget mellow yellow—a brighter shade is better.

—*Teen Vogue*, June/July 2004

Some Other Poetic Products:
Slime ball; Head wear; Hair pudding; Whipped Cream-Root Boost Mousse

African American women and other women with naturally curly hair.

Dealing with our locks can mean hairspray, gel, mousse, or whatever the latest hair goop is. While a new haircut can be a delightful transformation, it can also be a traumatic mistake we have to grow out. The notion of having a "bad hair day" has become a subject of conversation, an advertising theme, and an excuse not to face the world.

> A woman with cut hair is a filthy spectacle, and much like a monster; and all repute it a very great absurdity for a woman to walk abroad with shorn hair; for this is all one as if she should take upon her the form or person of a man, to whom short cut hair is proper.
>
> **–William Prynne, 1669 Puritan pamphlet**

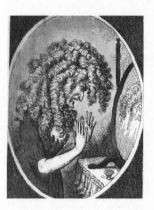

Having nice hair is something all girls are supposed to want, and just one more thing girls can get jealous about.

I like my hair, which is thin, long, a little wavy, and smooth; it feels soft. I use anti-frizz spray on it to school, to keep it flat and wear it like everyone else does, which is long and parted in the middle. At school it seems like having nice hair is something all girls are supposed to want, and just one more thing girls can get jealous about.

—Maggie, thirteen years old

I definitely think of hair as an accessory.

First I had dreads, then I had dreads on one side and shaved the other side. It was fun because I could still play with my hair and dye it cool colors. I definitely think of hair as an accessory. It's like clothing: Change it at will. My grandmother had a problem with it and said she wouldn't pay for me to go to college if I didn't shave off the dreads—she didn't approve of the fact that I couldn't comb my hair. So for her, having no hair at all was preferable.

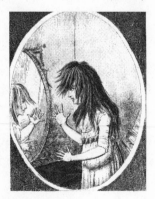

—Drew, seventeen years old

Shaving, Plucking, Waxing: The Battle over Body Hair

No one had heard of not shaving your legs.

In my old school, no one had heard of not shaving your legs, which was really strange to me. I almost started shaving my legs while I was there, but I didn't want to. Now I shave my armpits sometimes. A lot of people don't realize that you can shave for a long time and then just stop, no problem. One of my friends just started shaving her armpits—she finally gave in. I said, "Yeah, I used to do that, but I don't anymore." She was surprised and responded, "Really? You mean you can stop?"

—Rebecca, sixteen years old

Before 1915, hardly any women in the United States shaved their underarms and legs. Then, between 1915 and 1919, "The Great Underarm Campaign" in advertising began.[1] Ads told women that now that shorter dresses and sleeves were in fashion, body hair was "ugly," "unfashionable," and unclean.[2] The ads had a big impact. By 1945, the majority of women removed their leg and underarm hair, and these days 70 percent of American women use some type of hair removal technique.[3]

Outside of the pressure exerted by advertising, why do women shave their body hair? One theory is it makes the difference between men and women more obvious (a hairy guy, a smooth girl). Another is that shaving makes us look more childish—back to the days when we didn't have all that hair.[4] However, many cultures view body hair on women and men differently, and shaving goes in and out of fashion. In ancient Rome, women removed body hair with hot tar and razor-sharp shells.[5] Ouch! Many of today's European women let their underarm hair fly free, and it is seen as attractive. So decide for yourself if you want to shave or not—it grows back, so you can always decide again!

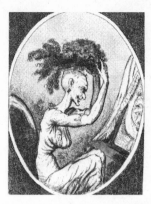

Having an afro or braids is a beautiful and easier alternative.

My mother always said, "Your hair is your tiara: All women must have nice hair, it makes you feminine." Being African American, the Western standards for hair, like soft and straight, are things that we don't naturally have. I used to spend three hours straightening my hair. But if I went out in the rain, it would be ruined. You become a slave to your hair. Having an afro or braids is a beautiful and easier alternative.

—Cassandra, eighteen years old

 Check out The African Pride Company for products designed to work with natural African American hair.

As we know, the top of the head is not the only place hair grows. The friendly follicles are all over our bodies, but congregate more densely in certain areas: armpits, pubic area, face, around the nipples, legs, forearms, that line straight down from the belly button, inside the nose, and on top of the big toe. Like hair on the head, body hair varies greatly from woman to woman. Some have the barely there, light, downy type of hair, while others have dark, heavy, prominent hair. The desirability of this hair is really up to the individual—just ask the bearded lady who chose to wear her long facial hair proudly.

Cosmetic Surgery and Procedures: Risky Business

I had my brows done once, decided I didn't like them, had the tattoo lasered off by a dermatologist, then redone by someone else. I even had a beauty mark tattooed by my eyebrow, and then I had that taken off. I have booked and then cancelled four nose jobs. My obsession has been time consuming and expensive . . . I have learned that my dissatisfaction with my appearance increases in direct proportion to how I feel.[7]

–Hope Donahue, who had seven plastic surgeries by the time she was twenty-seven and is the author of *Beautiful Stranger: A Memoir of an Obsession with Perfection*

Sixty million Americans have said that they don't like their noses, thirty million are unhappy with their chins, six million are displeased with their ears, and another six million don't dig their eyes.[8] These days, cosmetic surgery is being marketed as casually as a new fall wardrobe and Botox is being treated like a party favor. Thanks to TV shows that give us the play-by-plays of extreme makeovers and celebrities talking more openly about their "enhanced" body parts, there has been a boom of young people willing to go under the knife or have other invasive procedures. Botox injections (used mainly to reduce facial wrinkles) have increased by 133 percent among twenty- to thirty-nine-year-olds, and facelifts and chemical peels also rose dramatically since the makeover shows hit the air.[9] Botox treatments, which involve injecting a toxin that blocks nerves to paralyze the muscles that cause wrinkles, are costly and not without side effects. Short-term side effects include (depending on the area being treated): droopy eyelids, headache, nausea, and flu-like symptoms. Formal clinical evaluations of long-term Botox treatments have not been undertaken, yet women are still rushing to get these costly injections, which need to be repeated about every three months. Someone is smiling all the way to the bank, and probably not worrying about the laugh lines that smile is creating, either!

Plastic surgery is an aspect of surgery developed to correct deformities one may be born with (for example, a cleft lip) or may acquire (for example, scars from severe burns), and to restore function to the affected areas. Plastic surgery began in 200 BC in ancient India. Flaps of skin from the forehead were used to reconstruct women's noses that were mutilated by jealous husbands. Major strides were made during World War I, when plastic-surgery units were created to treat combat veterans injured on the front.

Cosmetic surgery is a branch of plastic surgery designed to improve or rejuvenate one's appearance. Benefiting from the knowledge gained from operating on wounded and burned soldiers and civilians, the practice of cosmetic surgery began after World War II. The most common procedures used to make a person look younger are face lifts, eyelid surgery, forehead lifts, and numerous body-tightening procedures, such as the tummy tuck and buttock and thigh lifts. Popular procedures to change one's looks are breast reductions and implants, nose jobs, and ear surgeries.

But just like makeup and clothes, cosmetic surgery can only change one's physical appearance. Our feelings about ourselves are only ours to change. Before considering cosmetic surgery, take a long look in the mirror and consider whether the change is worth spending thousands of dollars and facing the potential health risks (ranging from infections to death from anesthesia) associated with going under the knife. Ask yourself these questions:

1. Who wants the surgery? If it's not you, remember it is your body, not someone else's. You're the one who is going to have to live with it, so make the choice for yourself.
2. How realistic are your expectations? Keep in mind that no surgery will make you perfect or turn you into someone else.
3. How clear are you on the results you want? This is not about buying an expensive new sweater—it's a permanent change to your physical appearance.

Last year I had a nose job.

My mom made me feel like I needed to have a smaller nose, and I believed her. I didn't have expectations that it would change my life, which is good because it didn't. I think you have to go into it with realistic goals. A friend of mine also got a nose job, but she ended up with a tiny, tiny nose on her big face. She felt miserable. Now when I see people with big noses who are confident, I wonder why I couldn't have been like them.

—Taylor, eighteen years old

I've always felt like people should just get over it and like themselves the way they are.

I realize that's not really fair because I don't really have anything to get over. My friend who had a breast reduction operation said, "I know it will make my life easier, I'll be happier." I kind of wish she wouldn't have done it. There are some things I don't like about myself, but certainly nothing I could change with plastic surgery.

—Courtney, seventeen years old

Some people are happy and satisfied after a nose job, but some aren't because they expect too much.

My mom is a plastic surgeon. She says it's like being a psychiatrist because people come in with these problems that they think have to do with their appearance. Sometimes people think it will be a miraculous change. They think everyone will like them once their nose is different, but then they find something else that they don't like about themselves. If you feel like you have a big nose and it's really bothering you, get a nose job. If you feel better about yourself, great. Some people are happy and satisfied after a nose job, but some aren't because they expect too much. Some people don't like their new nose, it doesn't look good on them, and it takes them a long time to get used to it. It is permanent, so when you go in, you have to know what you are doing.

—Janet, seventeen years old

Rebelling: Trashing the Beauty Standard

Some of us are uncomfortable with the "pretty" mold and do everything to go against the norm. We boycott the Gap, shave our heads, pierce various body parts, tattoo ourselves, dress in whatever is not "in," or ditch the "nice girl" attitude. Rebelling against the beauty standard can be a statement that expresses our attitude about the world. Our body piercings and jet-black hair can say we don't care about looking like a fresh, young flower. Our green lipstick may be a way to separate ourselves from (or be accepted by) the gang. These days, an Izod shirt, loafers, and a quilted skirt can be our own form of rebellion. We may rebel to make a point or to express our inner emotions— or maybe we are just sick and tired of seeing the mainstream look.

I also wanted to destroy the possibility of looking beautiful.

I'm not your conventional Barbie doll/Miss America type. I shaved my head in January. I want people to know that I'm not trying to match their ideas of beauty, that I'm trying to match my own ideas of beauty. You know, girls are supposed to be pretty. I'm obsessed with beauty, and sometimes I think, "Oh, if I were beautiful like a model, everything would be great." Which is silly because I also don't want beauty to be the basis that people are judging me on. It scares me to look completely normal. In ninth grade I looked as strange as possible because I wanted people to know from the first that they couldn't judge me

An Image of Our Own

Tired of the same old fashion mags with their ever-changing list of beauty tips? Check out these cool alternatives (websites, too) that speak to us in real voices:

Adventure Divas

This TV program and website is about a group of divas too busy globe-trotting to focus on how they look in the mirror. There are documentaries of "adventure travel and modern-day heroines" set in Cuba, India, Iran, and more. www.adventuredivas.com

Adiosbarbie.com Ophira Edut created this site in 1999 to speak out against the impossible beauty standards we live with. She tells it straight and with a lot of humor. This website by the author of *Body Outlaws* is full of ideas and resources for dissing the mainstream media's idea of beauty and embracing the real diversity our world has to offer.
www.adiosbarbie.com

About-Face This San Francisco–based group combats negative and distorted images of women. Its mission is to promote positive self-esteem in girls and women of all ages, sizes, races, and backgrounds through a spirited approach to media education, outreach, and activism. "Through practical and activist methods we challenge our culture's overemphasis on physical appearance."
www.about-face.org

Bitch: Feminist Response to Pop Culture A print magazine devoted to "incisive commentary on our media driven world." Bitch offers critiques of TV, movies, and advertising along with interviews with "cool smart women" in all areas of pop culture.
www.bitchmagazine.com

Blue Jean A print magazine written and produced by young women (14–22), this is a great place to read true tales from peers and to submit your writing and artwork for a worldwide audience.
www.bluejeanonline.com

Just Think This organization was established in 1995 in response to facts like: "By age 18, the average American teenager will have spent more time watching television—25,000 hours—than learning in the classroom" (American Academy of Pediatrics). Like its title, this organization teaches young people to understand the words and images in media and to think for themselves.
www.justthink.org

Ms. First launched in 1971, this award-winning magazine was the first U.S. magazine to make feminist voices heard. Toss advice about having a bad hair day aside while you read expert coverage of issues relating to women's status, rights, and points of view.
www.msmagazine.com

ROCKRGRL Want to know about hip-hop feminists and influential all-female bands? This magazine "supports a woman's right to rock!" and has intelligent interviews with women in music—"because you're more than just a pretty face."
www.rockrgrl.com

Teen Voices Another publication that offers a place to submit your art and writing, this honest mag is "written by, for, and about teenage and adult women."
www.teenvoices.com

W.I.G. (Women in General) Focusing on women's worldwide culture, this website and magazine offers a place for women's "creativity, physicality, and ideas to shine in an open forum." www.wigmag.com

like they judge other girls. Then I grew up a little and thought, "Well, that's ridiculous." But it's still weird for me to walk down the street wearing jeans and a t-shirt looking like everyone else—I feel lost. In a lot of ways, that's bad because I should be confident enough about what's inside not to have to try and show it.

I hated high school. I was into this masochism thing because it's a quick release when you're feeling bad. I wanted to be beautiful all the time, but I also wanted to destroy the possibility of looking beautiful. I scratched my arms, and when my mom saw them, it was a big deal. So instead, I started piercing my ears. That was a more aesthetically pleasing way of destroying my body. I got my lip ring a week ago, and I like having it; it feels really good. I think it mirrors the chaos of moving from the suburbs to a new city. I feel like everything is kind of crazy, and this is something I can do to mark myself so I don't feel so lost.

—Tanya, seventeen years old

I like to wear strange clothes.

Everyone dresses in jeans and a shirt, but I like unusual, dark clothes, mostly black. My parents and some other people ask, "Did someone die? When is the funeral?" Ha ha. A lot of girls worry if other people like what they wear. I don't. If I like it, I get it.

—Theresa, fifteen years old

I went through my gothic stage in eighth grade.

I dyed my hair blue-black, wore really red lipstick and dark eyeliner. I decided I wanted to look unnatural. Then I dyed my hair fuchsia. For two years I went through pink, purple, whatever. Finally I dyed it back to black and let it grow out. It was fun, but then I got bored with it. People thought I was trying to make some big statement with it, but I was like, "No, I just think it's fun."

—Dina, eighteen years old

Putting Beauty in Its Place

What's on the outside isn't all there is.

It's not that how traditionally beautiful you are doesn't affect you at all. Certainly it does. If you are traditionally beautiful, what other people consider beautiful, then maybe it will seem like you have an easier time because people will want to be around you. But if you're beautiful and you have no thoughts of your own, people won't want to stay around you. And if you're not beautiful, but you do have thoughts of your own or you have a good character or if you have a great sense of humor or have interesting things to talk about, then eventually people are going to find you. I think that's part of growing up. People figure out, or I hope they figure out, that what's on the outside isn't all there is.

—Tara, sixteen years old

What if beauty were not such an important trait? If we were to grow up on a deserted island, we might always feel wonderful about how we looked, or we might not give it any thought. In our own isolated world, clothing might be worn just for warmth, pimples might be welcomed as beauty marks, and our own body type might symbolize perfection. Instead, we live in a world that tells us what is beautiful

Six Smart Tips to Be Media Savvy[10]

1. Step inside the minds of the media images: How do you think the people who construct the images that you see want you to feel? Realize that they might not have your best interests in mind; rather, they might solely have the intention of getting you to buy their product. If you are feeling insecure about how you look, you will be more likely to run to the store!

2. Do not believe that all the images you see are real. Lots of technology is used to reinvent reality. Remind yourself of the real people you love and respect.

3. Step back, listen to your gut reactions, and rationally evaluate image claims. Will your life really change with new sparkly lip gloss?

4. Do not fall into the trap of never-ending consumption. Part of the marketing game is to play on our vulnerability—to make us think that we need more stuff on the outside to feel good on the inside.

5. Identify media myths, such as "If I look perfect, I'll feel perfect."

6. Actively practice self-acceptance. Boost your own self-esteem so you can ignore all the cultural messages that can leave you feeling insufficient.

With a little practice, we can outsmart the media and not buy into the idea that we need to look a certain way to be happy.

and dictates that for girls, beauty is extremely important. Making things happen and living "happily ever after" is up to us, not our looks. We can take what we want from the beauty culture and throw out what makes us uncomfortable. Within the range of beauty possibilities, there is freedom to be ourselves. Check out page 33 for six tips on being media savvy. We need to find, create, and *insist* on valuing other images of beauty. Variety is the spice of life.

You shouldn't hurt yourself just to look a certain way.

Women in the media are perfect, thin people. But in real life, no one looks that perfect. You shouldn't hurt yourself just to look a certain way; not everyone can be tiny. Be true to yourself. Girls shouldn't have to be beautiful to impress men and be a guy's little creature. We should dress to impress ourselves.

—Zoe, eighteen years old

2

Body Image
Can't Get No Satisfaction?

nstead of smelling daisies or learning how to build boats, many of us spend our time focused on wishing and striving for the "perfect" body. Depending on the culture we grow up in, we may want to look like the tall and thin models in *Vogue* magazine or have the voluptuous curves of our favorite singer or actress. We may even take our quest for a better body to the extreme with crash diets, insane exercise regimens, and obsessive thoughts that are more harmful than beneficial.

Why isn't it that you eat what you want to stay healthy, exercise sometimes, and that's it?

Our society is obsessed with weight. Weight weight weight. A woman loses weight and says that's her best achievement ever. It's hard to stay sane in an atmosphere like our culture. Everything is low-fat, no-fat, diet this, low-carb that. All these women are trying to control their bodies. Separating your mind from your body is something that should be done with great care, yet this is done with great abandon: "I will not be hungry." So much concern over bodies has to do with growing older. Since now is a time of change for me and my friends, we're like, "I don't want to change drastically, I'm going to make my body do this or that." Controlling one's body is something that is possible, but dangerous.

—Robin, seventeen years old

People call me toothpick or washboard.

I wish I weren't so skinny. I want curves. I eat a lot, especially desserts—my dad calls me a bottomless pit. I can't seem to gain weight; I guess it's my metabolism. If I were more voluptuous, I think more guys would like me.

—Shawna, sixteen years old

I'm never critical of guys' bodies, though.

My mother always criticizes my body. She says, "You have nice hips and a thin waist, but your thighs are too muscular." She mentions a part of my body and then attaches a negative adjective to it. I find myself looking at other girls' body parts and criticizing them the way my mother does. I'm never critical of guys' bodies, though. Around girls, I wonder, "Wow, I never noticed she had cellulite," or "Gosh, she probably shouldn't be wearing that skirt." Then I go home and look at myself and think, "I wonder if that's what I look like, and what do they think of me?"

—Tara, sixteen years old

Thin, Thin, Thin: No Way to Win

We don't have to look far to see that our culture worships beauty and perfection in the form of a thin silhouette. Thin is everywhere: The woman on TV selling detergent is thin, the heroine in the latest blockbuster movie is definitely thin, and the fashion world is plagued with thinness. Magazines are full of articles on how to get the perfect butt in three weeks, trim your tummy, reduce cellulite, and firm your thighs. How can we be satisfied with our own sweet, round bellies or jiggling thighs amid all these messages? Many of us are fed up with this one-size body obsession and our "thin is in" culture. Aren't there more important things for us to be concerned with than looking perfect in jeans?

There is pressure for girls to be weaker, smaller versions of our full selves or to seek out an unnatural alteration to our natural, goddess-given forms. We need to stamp out the messages that say women's bodies should look a certain way or not take up space, and rejoice in our strength and in our *natural* body shapes. The world is full of diversity. Nature celebrates these differences—shouldn't we?

Going . . . going . . . gone?

There is a lot of brainpower being focused on how our bodies look (or don't look):

☀ In a study of fifth graders, ten-year-old girls and boys told researchers they were dissatisfied with their own bodies after watching a music video by Britney Spears or a clip from the TV show *Friends*.[1]

☀ By age thirteen, 53 percent of American girls are "unhappy with their bodies." This dissatisfaction increases to 78 percent by the time girls reach seventeen.[2]

☀ Teenage girls who viewed commercials depicting women who modeled the unrealistically thin ideal of beauty felt less confident, angrier, and more dissatisfied with their weight and appearance afterward.[3]

No wonder we are unhappy with our own bodies and so many of us want to be thinner—the women depicted in the media have been shrinking over time:

☀ Since 1959, the average weight of Miss America has decreased twenty-five pounds, while the average height has increased three inches. Forty years ago, the average Miss America wore a size ten dress. Today, the average is a size two![4]

☀ Between 1959 and 1979, *Playboy* centerfolds steadily declined in weight to reach their current unrealistically thin level.

☀ During the past eighty-five years, young girls depicted in children's textbooks have become thinner and thinner.

☀ In 1893, the executives of the White Rock Company purchased the trademark rights to a painting by Paul Thurman of Psyche, the goddess of purity, and made her the White Rock Girl. Over the years, the Psyche image on the White Rock beverage labels became longer legged, slimmer hipped, and more streamlined.[5] Her figure changed from an estimated five feet, four inches tall and 140 pounds in 1894 to her current five feet, ten inches tall and 110 pounds.[6]

	1894	1947	1970
HEIGHT	5'4"	5'6"	5'8"
NECK	12.5"	12.5"	12"
BUST	37"	35"	35"
WAIST	27"	25"	24"
HIPS	38"	35"	34"
THIGH	22.5"	20.5"	19.5"
KNEE	15"	14"	13"
CALF	13.2"	13"	12"
ANKLE	7.4"	8"	7.5"
WEIGHT	140 lbs.	125 lbs.	110 lbs.

The White Rock Girl: from left to right are the measurements for 1894, 1947, and 1970

The Incredible Shrinking Woman

☀ It is hard to believe these days, but for most of history, the ideal body shape for women was plump and round. Eating all the food you wanted was a luxury for the wealthy, so extra weight represented a higher place in society. This plumper ideal still exists in many cultures, but thanks to our media, American culture has worshipped thinness for the past thirty-five years.

Though the trend has been from plump to thin, the path has not been straight. The ideal body standard has bounced around dramatically. Over the past century, we've gone from plump to thin, to voluptuous, back to thin, then to thin with muscle tone. It is amazing how we are influenced by a beauty standard that varies like the weather.

☀ In the 1920s, when the look for the "modern" woman was boyish and sleek and women's clothing became much more revealing, there was a surge of eating disorders and exercise fads among women.

☀ During the Depression (the 1930s), our culture became more traditional in its values, and a rounder woman returned as the ideal.

☀ In the 1950s, sex sirens were in and we needed a body like an hourglass, à la Marilyn Monroe.

☀ In the 1960s, when the women's movement was making strides toward equality, a skinny, boyish figure like Twiggy's became the ideal.

☀ In the 1980s, it was important to have a skinny figure, but now with the muscle tone of an athlete. Big breasts also made a comeback, so many women rushed to cosmetic surgeons for implants.

☀ In the 1990s, while there was still an emphasis on muscle tone and cleavage, the frail waif and the spaced-out, scrawny, "heroin" models elbowed their way onto the fashion pages.

☀ In the 2000s, sex appeal is popularly defined as thin yet shapely. Even when we are pregnant or aging, it's all about having a "hot" body. More women go under the knife than ever before.

Is It Time to Recycle Some of Those Magazines?

Girls in grades 5-12 were asked how often they read women's fashion magazines and how this influenced them. Some 69 percent reported that the appearance of models in the magazines influenced their image of a perfect female body, and 47 percent desired to lose weight because of the magazine pictures. Frequent readers of women's fashion magazines (two to seven times a week) were more likely to have dieted or exercised to lose weight because of a magazine article.[1]

The more I see girls who are too thin, the less I want to look like them. I want a body.

These models look like little girls who don't eat enough—it's not natural at all. At an age when you are looking for affirmation, you are supposed to worry about your body. In our society, a woman's body is supposed to fit a man's ideal. I hate to blame society for the injustices that have been done to me, though—I think that is silly. Most is from yourself and your family. It's about control. The girls I know who don't eat want to control what is going on in their life.

—Helen, sixteen years old

I was torn between two cultures.

In my culture you have to be sort of plump. But I was very skinny growing up. From fifteen to seventeen, my mom gave me six pills a day to enhance my appetite. But now, when I look at those pictures, I was plump! I was bigger than I am now, but for the Haitian people, I was too skinny. Then when I came here to college, skinny was good. My roommates would tell me, "Let's try to lose weight," or "Let's go and work out." Then when I would go back to Haiti, my family would say, "Are you starving to death there? You look horrible, you look terrible." Being torn between these two cultures, I never knew where I should be.

—Marie, eighteen years old

My body is thin naturally.

Sometimes people get paranoid because I'm really thin. Some girls put me down or say, "Oh, she's just thin because she has an eating disorder, she exercises all the time, and she must put her whole life into looking that way." I have to be careful and walk around those subjects, or people put me in a category. I hear girls all around me say "I'm so fat," and they're not. I explain that my body is thin naturally, that's the way my whole family is—it's hereditary. I don't know if they believe me, though.

—Angie, seventeen years old

Not all of us idealize a skinny body. We need to listen to those of us who have strong defenses against the "thin is the only way to win" message.

Either heard or taught
as girls
we thought
that skinny was funny
or a little bit
silly
and feeling a pull
toward the large and the colorful
I would joke you
when
you grew too thin.

But your new kind of hunger
makes me chilly
like danger
for I see you forever retreating
shrinking
into a stranger
in flight—
and
growing up
black and fat
I was so sure
that skinny
was funny
or silly
but always
white.

—Audre Lorde, "Song for a Thin Sister," *Undersong*

I have a kind of typical Cuban body, which means a small chest and large hips.

When I was taking ballet, I would have to squeeze and tuck my butt all the time to try to fit the "right" ballerina figure—it was terrible and could not have been good for my body. Now I take more modern dance and I feel freer to be who I am.

—Lucia, nineteen years old

We find ideals outside of the white model scene.

Black women are usually bigger than the skinny ideal and have less messed-up attitudes about their body image. My friends (who are black) have role models who aren't skinny—like Lil' Kim the rap artist, who's slender but not bony, and Queen Latifah, who's big and classy. Since YM and Seventeen are like 90 percent white, there's less to relate to and compare ourselves to, so we find ideals outside of the white model scene.

—Kimra, fourteen years old

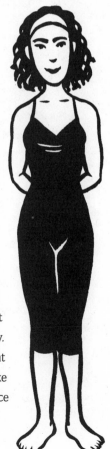

Dieting and Exercise: Are We Out of Control?

In a national survey of nine- and ten-year-old girls, 40 percent have already attempted to lose weight.[2] This is not because at age ten we suddenly become fat. Actually, a very small proportion of nine- to ten-year-old girls are overweight. So why do so many of us try to lose weight? Because we are told that being thinner will change our lives. The perfect body supposedly offers success, love, control, and stability, and dieting has been sold to us as the key to our success. The additional emphasis on muscle tone and fit bodies makes us feel as if we should be on a rigid, intense workout schedule, battling every bulge. There is a cultural fascination with "before and after" stories of people who have lost weight and re-sculpted themselves to look more magazine-friendly. The screaming headlines draw us in: "I lost forty pounds in eight weeks, got new boobs, and now I laugh at my ex-boyfriend." It's like a fairy tale with a happy ending, but instead of marrying Prince Charming, the princess is able to wear a size eight dress and show off cellulite-free legs and more cleavage.

In my head, I knew I didn't need to lose weight.

You want to say to a friend who is dieting like crazy, "Are you okay? Is something wrong? Why are you doing this?" But they don't want to hear that from you. In my town, appearance is the number-one important thing. Starting in middle school, all the girls diet and feel like they have to work out. It affected me, even though in my head I knew I didn't need to lose weight. I have a friend who would eat only a baked potato and a bagel all day. That is ridiculous. I don't think my friends need to worry about their weight. They complain, "I'm so fat," but none of them are.

—Sonia, seventeen years old

Real Bodies: Loving the One You Have

Check out these books which confront America's obsession with thinness:

Am I Thin Enough Yet? The Cult of Thinness and the Commercialization of Identity by Sharlene Hesse-Biber, Oxford: Oxford University Press, 1997.

The Body Project: An Intimate History of American Girls by Joan Jacobs Brumberg, New York: Vintage, 1998.

Body Outlaws: Rewriting the Rules of Beauty and Body Image edited by Ophira Edut, Emeryville, CA: Seal Press, 2003.

Bountiful Women: Large Women's Secrets for Living the Life They Desire by Bonnie Bernell, Berkeley, CA: Wildcat Canyon Press, 2000.

The Fat Girls Guide to Life by Wendy Shanker, New York: Bloomsbury, 2004.

Fat History: Bodies and Beauty in the Modern West by Peter N. Stearns, New York: New York University Press, 2002.

Fat Is a Feminist Issue by Susie Orbach, New York: Galahad Books, 1997.

FAT!SO?: Because You Don't Have to Apologize for Your Size by Marilyn Wann, Berkeley, CA: Ten Speed Press, 1998.

The Best Kept Secret: Diets Don't Work

"I've tried Slim Fast and Atkins and each time I lost weight but then had uncontrollable cravings and I gained the weight right back."

—Karina, seventeen years old

Advertisements for weight-loss programs or products promise great results. However, only about 5 to 10 percent of dieters are able to successfully lose weight and *maintain* that loss, something the $1.7 billion-per-year weight-loss industry never tells us.[3]

So why are we likely to be failed dieters? Simple—the desire to get thin by

The Invisible Woman: Confronting Weight Prejudice in America by W. Charisse Goodman, Carlsbad, CA: Gürze Books, 1995.

Love the Body You Were Born With: A Ten-Step Workbook for Women by Monica Dixon, New York: Berkley Publishing Group, 1996.

Minding the Body: Women Writers on Body and Soul edited by Patricia Foster, New York: Doubleday, 1994.

No Fat Chicks: How Big Business Profits by Making Women Hate Their Bodies—and How to Fight Back by Terry Poulton, Secaucus, NJ: Carol Publishing Group, 1997.

Nothing to Lose: A Guide to Sane Living in a Larger Body by Cheri K. Erdman, San Francisco: Harper, 1995.

The Obsession: Reflections on the Tyranny of Slenderness by Kim Chernin, New York: HarperPerennial Library, 1994.

Self-Esteem Comes in All Sizes: How to Be Happy and Healthy at Your Natural Weight by Carol A. Johnson, Carlsbad, CA: Gürze Books, 2001.

Shadow on a Tightrope: Writings by Women on Fat Oppression edited by Lisa Schoenfielder and Barb Wieser, San Francisco: Aunt Lute Books, 1983.

Wake Up, I'm Fat! by Camryn Manheim, New York: Broadway Books, 2000.

limiting food intake makes no sense to our bodies. Extreme changes in our diet can make us irritable, depressed, or sluggish. And our metabolic rate slows—that is, we burn fewer calories—as we diet because our bodies are designed to help us survive food shortages. With regular exercise and balanced, nutritious meals, we can maintain a healthy, fit body (see sidebar "An Alternative to Dieting: Healthy Eating" on pages 50–51).

Diets that create imbalance because they are restrictive or extreme lead to food obsessions and episodes of overeating. When we diet in this way, we deprive our body of calories and nutrients, so that when we go off the diet, we tend to overeat. Those foods we don't allow ourselves to eat during a diet may become even more tempting. We also adopt the unhealthy attitude that being "good" means eating only allowable or "good" foods, while any departure into off-limit foods makes us "bad." Restrictive dieting sets us up to feel guilty.

Taking Our Bodies to the Extreme: How Much Is Too Much?

Even when I felt sick, I'd exercise for the whole hour.

I used to exercise for an hour every day. I usually used a stationary bike at the gym. The sweat would pour down my face, and I would keep pushing myself harder and harder until I felt sick. Even when I felt sick, I'd do it for the whole hour—I'd watch the clock and count down the minutes until I could stop. If I didn't exercise for one hour, I would feel uncomfortable in my body the whole day. It has only been recently that I feel less guilty about not exercising and don't have to do it every day.

—Lynn, seventeen years old

This obsession isn't seen as the disease it is.

You will never have a supermodel body and keep it if you weren't born that way. It's a myth that's so ingrained in our society, and people are feeling bad because they don't look a certain way and they feel like they are failing. If you feel like a failure because you are not a certain weight, that says a lot about our society. It's not your fault. I do hold society and the media responsible for a lot of my own body concerns. Extreme dieting is condoned, even admired by people. The fact that girls think it would be cool to eat one apple a day is scary. This obsession isn't seen as the disease it is until girls on extreme diets end up in the hospital. An eating disorder doesn't have to be anorexia, bulimia, or compulsive overeating. An eating

disorder includes extreme dieting and means the way you eat is "not in order."
A lot of people think, "I'm just on a diet," but it's a lot more than that.

—Rebecca, seventeen years old

How do we know when a diet or a fitness regimen has gone too far? If a diet is making us feel faint and food is the focus of our lives, it's too extreme. If we exercise because we want to mold our body into a completely different shape, and we feel worthless if we don't meet our goals, then we've lost perspective. The following are warning signs for obsessive exercising and dieting:

- We spend most of our free time engaged in or thinking about dieting or exercise.
- Our emotional investment in dieting or exercise is greater than our investment in school, friends, or family.
- Our period stops because of weight loss from dieting.
- We exercise past the point when our body says to stop, and we exercise even when we are injured.

How much we are exercising or how few calories we are consuming may become the basis for our self-image: "Today I totally avoided sugar—I'm doing so well," or "I can't believe I ate a second piece of chocolate cake—I'm a miserable slob." This kind of thinking may be a way of avoiding the real problems or stresses in our lives. Confronting the deeper issues can put dieting and exercise into proper perspective. For some helpful resources on facing our emotions rather than attacking our shape and weight, see the sidebar on pages 42–43.

If you think you may be obsessively dieting or exercising, please read the next chapter on eating disorders, which gives resources for dealing with this behavior.

Body Dysmorphic Disorder

Body dys . . . what? Body dysmorphic disorder (or BDD for short) is when dissing our bodies becomes an obsession and a psychological condition. BDD is serious and is growing quickly in our culture: about one out of every fifty people experiences BDD, and most who do are in their teens or twenties. If we suffer from BDD, we not only dislike some aspect of how we look, but we also become preoccupied to the point that we think of nothing else and have a hard time being seen by others without focusing on our flaws. And these "flaws" are either imagined by us or are based only on a slight imperfection that we blow way out of proportion. Any body part can be the focus of concern, but most often it is the skin, hair, nose, or ears. We may have BDD if we show some of the following symptoms:

- We check ourselves in the mirror over and over.
- Or the opposite—we avoid mirrors.
- We avoid having our picture taken.
- We wear camouflage to cover up our imagined flaws.
- We groom ourselves excessively.
- We pick at our skin to make it smooth.
- We touch the "defect" and even measure it repeatedly.
- We constantly request reassurance about our imagined defect.
- We make repeated medical visits to get rid of our imagined flaw.

Some people with BDD are able to deal well with daily life; however, some can be paralyzed by the symptoms and experience depression, anxiety, and a desire to avoid social situations altogether. What helps: To date, cognitive behavioral therapy or behavioral modification therapy and certain medications have been effective for those with body dysmorphic disorder.[4] What does *not* help? Cosmetic surgery.

For more information on BDD, check out *The Broken Mirror: Understanding and Treating Body Dysmorphic Disorder* by Katharine Phillips, MD (Oxford: Oxford University Press, 1998) and *The BDD Workbook: Overcome Body Dysmorphic Disorder and End Body Image Obsessions* by James Claiborn and Cherry Pedrick (Oakland, CA: New Harbinger, 2002).

Self-Injury (Cutting)

You have so much pain inside yourself that you try to hurt yourself on the outside.

—**Princess Diana** (admitting in a television interview
that she intentionally cut her arms and legs)

Self-injury is another extreme assault on our bodies. It is the practice of purposefully harming ourselves in the hopes of temporarily blocking our mental or emotional pain, such as guilt, rejection, anxiety, boredom, and chaotic or obsessive thoughts. Cutting is the most common form of self-injury, but other forms include: head banging, hitting, burning the skin, picking at scabs or wounds to prevent healing, and even breaking bones on purpose. The infliction of pain is a way of taking our minds off feelings or thoughts that we would rather not experience. According to surveys of self-injurers, the average person who self-mutilates is female and usually begins this behavior at age fourteen.[5]

Treatment for self-injury often involves working with a counselor and unlearning the self-injury behavior by keeping an impulse-control log and journal to help sort through the urge to injure oneself. This type of therapy can help us deal directly with what is really making us upset, sad, anxious, numb, or depressed. Finding an outlet for our pain and emotions is key, and may involve writing, drawing, and getting involved in other forms of creativity. The following is a list of symptoms that may indicate that we (or someone we know) need help:[6]

- We obsess about hurting ourselves.
- We sometimes can't explain where our injuries come from.
- We get anxious when our wounds start to heal.
- We often believe that if we don't self-injure, we'll go crazy or explode.
- We figure that no one can hurt us more than we can hurt ourselves.
- We can't imagine life without self-injury.
- If we stop self-injuring, we think our parents win.
- We often self-injure as a way to punish ourselves.
- We often self-injure to show others how we feel.
- We almost always carry something with us that we can use to self-injure.

For more information on self-injury, we can call the SAFE Alternative Program at (800) DONT-CUT (366-8288) or go to www.selfinjury.com. Read *Cutting: Understanding and Overcoming Self-Mutilation* by Steven Levenkron (New York: W. W. Norton, 1998), or *A Bright, Red Scream* by Marilee Strong (New York: Penguin USA, 1999). Also check out *The Cutting Edge*, a newsletter by and for women who self-mutilate, PO Box 20819, Cincinnati, OH 44120.

Eating and Self-Image

It's hard to enjoy food if we're worried others are judging us by what and how much we eat. The fun of eating with others is shattered if we are paranoid that all eyes are on our plate. Instead of questioning why anyone would care if we eat another Oreo cookie, a bag of chips, or a platter of tofu, we sometimes assume that it will be viewed as a character flaw. We become hyperaware of imaginary rules: Don't eat as much as a boy, don't eat junk food, eat what everyone else is eating, don't eat another helping. Consider this: People are probably thinking about their next class or are busy scanning the cafeteria rather than noticing how many bites we have taken. Food should be nourishing, not anxiety-provoking!

My boyfriend loved me no matter what I looked like.

Before I met my boyfriend, I wouldn't eat all day until dinner at eight o'clock. At the end of the school day, when we had math, I couldn't concentrate at all. Then I would eat a ton at dinner. When I would go out on a date, I would eat a salad, and the guy would be eating a hamburger or a steak and fries. After a few dates with my boyfriend, I ate more like him. I've gained weight, but I don't care. My boyfriend gave me confidence—he really loved me no matter what I looked like. He saw me in sweats and everything. Growing up, we get the message that boys are supposed to be physically strong and girls are supposed to be weak. I think that affects our eating habits.

—Letitia, seventeen years old

My friends started calling me the "tofu princess."

After reading Fast Food Nation, *I started changing my diet to eat more macrobiotic with lots of veggies and whole grains and less meat and junk food. My energy was great as a result and I felt really clearheaded, but the hard thing was that my friends started making fun of me and calling me "the tofu princess." It's not that I won't eat sugar anymore, I mean I still have my soft spot for brownies, but I like knowing how different foods affect me . . . that what is going into my body is becoming me! So I've learned to smile when they tease me. And if I'm at a pizza party and I feel like eating the pizza because it makes me feel connected then I'll eat it, but then I go back to my kale and quinoa. That's me.*

—Jessica, eighteen years old

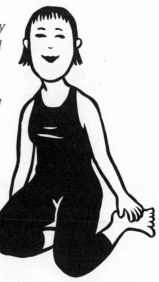

In public I'm more nibbly.

Sometimes when I'm around people I don't know, I'm not as comfortable eat-ing. If I'm hanging out with my friends at home, we'll eat anything, be gross, and it doesn't matter. But in public I'm more nibbly and eat less, to seem more polite. The guys I know always seem comfortable, they just dig right in.

—Maria, seventeen years old

I don't alter my eating habits.

A lot of my friends just eat salads when they are out on dates. I don't alter my eating habits at all around my boyfriend; I'm comfortable with him. If I'm hungry, I'll get more. I don't think, "One more piece of pizza, how horrible." If I didn't eat when I was hungry, I'd make myself miserable.

—Aiko, seventeen years old

How to Get Fit and Still Have a Life

What is a healthy way to get in shape? For one thing, the quick fixes don't work. Crash diets and extreme exercising only lead to burnout and disappointment when the weight returns. To successfully achieve and maintain a healthy body, we need to incor-porate moderate exercise and good nutrition into our routine. Here are some approaches that will keep both our body and our mind healthy:

- Don't focus on weight; focus on health and fitness.
- Exercise can involve anything from walking up stairs or taking long walks to working out or competing on an athletic team.
- Eating healthy means getting in tune with our appetite and feeding ourselves when we are hungry.
- Counting calories is not the solution. A healthy alternative is to eat more fruits, vegetables, and grains, and to lower our intake of fats, meats, and sweets.
- We shouldn't freak out if we sometimes eat when we are not hungry, or if we eat more "junk" than we planned on. Feeling guilty doesn't help.
- Cutting back on fat can be good, but we should not let it interfere with our life. Remember, our body needs some fat.

An Alternative to Dieting: Healthy Eating

Diets don't work because they deprive us and deny our body the nutrients it may need in order to grow and keep us healthy. With a diet, we follow a set of instructions and directions. With healthy eating, we simply tune in to our body and listen to what it is telling us it requires.

The following are thoughts and suggestions from Sigi Weiss of www.bodily wisdom.com on how to create healthy habits (and it's not all about food!):

❊ Drink plenty of pure water throughout the day, and reduce your intake of sugary and caffeinated beverages, which affect both mood and blood-sugar levels.

❊ Add movement or exercise into your daily life. Don't be a couch potato and sit in front of the television or computer all day. Try something new: competitive sports, a yoga or dance class, hiking, or just dancing in your room. Just keep moving. Even small amounts of exercise throughout the day can benefit your health.

❊ Make any changes to your eating habits gradually and subtly. Avoid making drastic changes overnight.

❊ Instead of giving up certain foods, add healthy choices (more whole grains, fresh vegetables, and fruits) to what you are already eating. Over time, you will "crowd out" the junk food with the healthier choices.

❊ Explore new foods. Go shopping with your friends, parents, or siblings. See what's out there, and get curious. You can pick a new veggie, fruit, or grain each week, bring it home, and try a recipe.

❊ Add color to your diet. Eat colorful things—red, orange, yellow, and green. And we don't mean candy! We are talking about nature's colorful fruits and vegetables—each color offers different nutrients.

❊ Don't skip meals or fast. When you skip meals, your blood sugar goes down and you feel exhausted, and the next thing you know, you want to eat everything in sight.

❄ Make time for breakfast. Breakfast starts your metabolism off for the day. A good breakfast helps you to think better and gives you more energy.

❄ Sleep at least eight hours a night. Teens are sleep-deprived because they often stay up late and then have to wake up early for school. This negatively affects the nervous system and changes our appetite patterns.

❄ Take time off. We can always be on the run with school and extracurricular activities. We need time out to do nothing. Meditation is a great tool for tuning in to yourself. Look at an object (like a leaf) for five to ten minutes, and notice all the details.

❄ Be social. Don't isolate yourself. If you feel lonely or sad, get a snuggle from a parent, pet, or friend.

❄ Make good choices with friends. Make two lists of friends: people that you like, and those who drain your energy. Try to take a break from the ones who make you feel down or stressed out. Having only one or two friends who make you feel good about yourself is better than having ten who make you miserable.

❄ Keep a journal. Write down your thoughts. Writing can be a great outlet.

The more we can focus on our health and positive qualities instead of fussing over our weight, the healthier we will be. Here are some websites that can help us explore new healthy eating habits:

www.teenshealth.org/teen/recipes/

www.whfoods.com/cookhealthy.php

www.wholefoodsmarket.com/recipes/index.html

www.integrativenutrition.com/recipes.asp

If we could just relax and not take diets, eating, or exercise to an extreme, we would probably be a lot happier. So throw away those crazy diets and quick-fix books! Remember that impossible exercise standards defeat the purpose that exercise should lower stress, not cause it. If we feel out of control about our eating or exercising, talking to a counselor may help us understand what is going on.

Women in Sports

Although these days athletic women are considered cool, this wasn't always the case. In the Victorian period, the ideal female was "passive, frail, delicate, ethereal, and soft."[1] Women were told that exercise was bad for them, that it would affect their ability to have babies, and that their bodies were not made to handle the stress. While menstruating, women weren't supposed to engage in any physical activity and were sometimes confined to bed.

Traditionally, men competed in sports and women cheered on the sidelines. In the mid-1800s, acceptable recreational activities for American women were limited to croquet, horseback riding, archery, and ice skating. By the late 1800s, some women were playing tennis and golf. The first team and contact sport for women was basketball (1892), but it was controversial and each player was restricted to playing only one-third of the court! Here's a look at some highlights in women's sports:[2]

1928 After much struggle, five women's track-and-field events are added to the male-dominated Olympics.

1948 Alice Coachman becomes the first African American woman to win an Olympic gold medal (high jump).

1963 Volleyball is introduced as the first team sport for women in the Olympic Games.

1967 Disguised as a man, Katherine Switzer is the first woman to run the Boston Marathon.

1973 Billie Jean King defeats Bobby Riggs in a tennis match publicized as the "Battle of the Sexes." King has won more Wimbledon titles than any other tennis player, male or female.

☼ We might want to educate ourselves with a good book on nutrition, like *Healing With Whole Foods: Asian Traditions and Modern Nutrition* by Paul Pitchford (Berkeley, CA: North Atlantic Books, 2002), *The Wellness Encyclopedia of Food and Nutrition* (New York: Random House, 1992), *Nourishing Wisdom: A Mind/ Body Approach to Nutrition and Well-Being* by Marc David (New York: Bell Tower, 1994), or *Food and Healing* by Annemarie

1988 Sarah Fulcher finishes the longest continuous solo run ever in her 11,134-mile run around the perimeter of the United States. She ran for fourteen months, averaging a marathon a day.

1990 Susan Butcher wins her fourth Alaskan 1,049-mile Iditarod Trail Dog Sled Race.

1997 Two professional women's basketball leagues are formed—the ABL (American Basketball League) and the WNBA (Women's National Basketball Association).

1999 Mia Hamm breaks the international scoring record for women and men's soccer with her 108th career goal. The success of the U.S. Women's Soccer team creates a boom for girls' and women's soccer.

2002 Tennis icons Venus and Serena Williams' performances in the French Open make them the number one and number two players in the world—a first for siblings and a breakthrough for African American women in tennis.

There is a revolution in women's sports going on in the United States, thanks in large part to Title IX of the Educational Amendments—way cool legislation passed in 1972 prohibiting sex discrimination in education programs and helping to create tons of opportunities for girls in school sports. As a result, girls today are more likely to learn that it's okay to be strong and competitive—characteristics that lead to success in athletics and in life. Recent studies are trumpeting the news that athletic girls have greater academic success and higher self-esteem as well.

Colbin (New York: Ballantine, 1996). Or check out books that blow the cover off the diet and food industries, like Laura Fraser's *Losing It: America's Obsession With Weight and the Industry That Feeds On It* (New York: Dutton, 1997) and Eric Schlosser's *Fast Food Nation: The Dark Side of the All-American Meal* (New York: Perennial, 2002).

Exercise clears my head.

I exercise, but I don't feel pressure to do it. I jog, and I used to swim. Exercise clears my head and helps me to mentally relax, like when I've been writing a paper all day. I listen to my Walkman, and it's nice to be by myself. I also take kickboxing, for fun and for self-defense. In general, being physically strong builds my self-confidence.

—Zoe, sixteen years old

I lost weight without dieting, binging, or purging.

Girls need to get the right information and not get fooled by some ads to replace meals with shakes—you can't keep that up! I put on a lot of weight a few years ago, and kids were cruel to me. Finally a close friend asked why I had blown up, and that's when I decided to ask my doctor for advice. He told me to cut way down on the junk that I was eating—I used to eat fries, hamburgers, and chips every day. Now I just eat those foods occasionally, and I eat a lot more vegetables and fruits. My weight went down slowly to a more comfortable level and remains stable. Common sense does work!

—Maxine, fifteen years old

Being Overweight: It's Not a Crime

.It is important that you exercise control when you eat . . . . Don't let your heart take over. Eat like a human being, not a fat person.
—Judy Mazel, *The Beverly Hills Diet*

What? So fat people are not human beings? This is an example of the outrageous way overweight people are sometimes treated. Young kids tease heavier kids and call them "ugly," "lazy," or "sloppy." As people get older, "unhappy" and "weak-willed" are added to the list. These stereotypes are ridiculous. Our weight doesn't dictate who we are.

We are bombarded by conflicting messages: Ads screaming at us to buy two double-deluxe burgers for the price of one, or to take another slice of "sinfully" delicious ice cream cake, are followed by ads urging us to join the growing number of women who have lost fifty pounds on the newest "amazing" diet plan, or telling us to eat Special K so we can be like the thin-thighed woman who can now fit into those super-skinny jeans. This media schizophrenia—equating joy in life with eating high-calorie junk food *and* being skinny—may make those of us who are overweight feel not only frustrated but also guilty and ashamed of our bodies.

It's all about self-confidence.

My big cover-up for everything was being an individual—I had purple hair; I was the big punk. I wasn't "Thin Tina" or "Fat Tina," I was just "Tina." I gained about fifty pounds in the ninth grade. It just sort of happened. Now I'm gradually losing it. I don't think diets work, and they are not healthy. I've lost thirteen pounds over the last three months just by walking a lot. I'm not doing it to look like everyone else; I'm doing it because I want to do it. I don't set restrictions; I eat whatever I want and know that I will walk for a mile so it will all work out.

I don't feel sorry for people who want to be skinny; I think it's ridiculous and humorous. They are obviously not happy with themselves. They should fix what's in

The Fat Liberation Movement

In the 1970s, the fat liberation movement began among women who were questioning and protesting our society's prejudices about fat people—sizism. Referring to the atmosphere we live in as "fat oppression", this movement speaks out against our society's ridiculous standards for beauty and its rejection of fat people, and emphasizes self-love and acceptance of all body types.

My body is fucking beautiful, and every time I look in the mirror and acknowledge that, I am contributing to the revolution.

—Nomy Lamm, *"It's a Big Fat Revolution"*

their head, not their body, because otherwise they will never be happy. If you are vomiting, or starving, or eating fatty foods all day long, that's a problem. But if you are heavier than another person, I don't see the problem. It's all about self-confidence. I'm big, but I've always been happy with myself. The people who judge other people's appearance are not happy with themselves. If someone has to go around insulting or commenting on people's bodies, they must be unhappy. I don't feel that need.

—Tina, seventeen years old

I just have a different body type; it's not about what I eat.

By the age of ten, I realized that my body was naturally bigger than most of my friends'. I just have a different body type; it's not about what I eat. I can eat less than my friend Suzy, and I'll still always weigh more than she does. My parents are pretty hefty, and I know I will always be too. Two years ago I tried the dieting thing, but I was always hungry and I started to think about food all the time. Now, I exercise when I'm in the mood and have gotten more comfortable with my shape. My friends love me the way I am, not for how much I weigh.

—Lena, sixteen years old

Food for me is so comforting, and a kind of escape, but I'm working on dealing with my feelings.

I eat when I'm depressed, bored, angry, or sad, which is a whole lot of the time. I know I'm too big and it's unhealthy, but that just makes me feel worse, so I eat more. I started going to Overeaters Anonymous, which has helped me realize my own tendencies, and I realize I am not alone. Food for me is so comforting, and a kind of escape, but I'm working on dealing with my feelings. It's not about fitting into a size ten anymore, it's about feeling complete without feeling stuffed, and loving myself.

—Gilda, seventeen years old

It's estimated that one-third of Americans could be defined as "obese," that is, 20 percent over the ideal body weight for their age and height. There are health risks associated with being obese, including high blood pressure and a greater likelihood of developing adult-onset diabetes. We should be aware, however, that charts giving ideal body weights are not always accurate, especially if they do not consider our height. Also, the true basis for determining obesity is our percentage of body fat, not our weight. This means it is possible to be fit and fat, and that a healthy lifestyle is more important than what the scale tells us.[7]

Where the Fat Girls Are—and Proud of It!

Check out these organizations and publications that promote fat-positive attitudes:

Fat!So? For People Who Don't Apologize for Their Size

A witty, upbeat magazine and website, complete with Aunt Agony's advice column and fat-positive t-shirts and posters. PO Box 423464, San Francisco, CA 94142, phone: (800) OH-FATSO, email: marilyn@fatso.com, website: www.fatso.com

International Size Acceptance Association

Its mission is to promote size acceptance and fight size discrimination throughout the world by means of advocacy and action. Its website has links to other size-wise organizations as well as a link for teens. PO Box 82126, Austin, TX 78758, email: teenpals@size-acceptance.org, website: www.size-acceptance.org

National Association to Advance Fat Acceptance

NAAFA is a non-profit organization, founded in 1969, that works to eliminate discrimination based on body size and to provide people with the tools for self-empowerment through public education, advocacy, and member support. PO Box 188866, Sacramento, CA 95818, email: naafa@naafa.org, website: www.naafa.org

Radiance: The Magazine for Large Women

A glossy, colorful magazine with articles on health, the media, fashion, and politics. phone: (510) 885-1505, website: www.radiancemagazine.com

Sizewise

An online resource for clothing, products, fat-positive organizations, and more. website: www.sizewise.com

Breasts: They Come in All Shapes and Sizes

Most women don't know what "normal" breasts look like. Most of us haven't seen many other women's breasts, and have been constantly exposed since childhood to the "ideal" image of breasts that permeates our society. But few of us fit that image, and there's no reason why we should. The range and size of breasts is so wide that it's hard to say what's "normal."

-Susan M. Love, MD, *Dr. Susan Love's Breast Book*

A Mini History of Breasts in America

1920s   Women bound their breasts tightly to create the flat-chested, boyish flapper look.

1950s   Marilyn Monroe and Jane Russell rendered the flat chest unattractive. Women wore padded, underwired, push-up bras to make the most of whatever they had.

1960s   Super skinny models like Twiggy made the flat chest fashionable again.

1970s   Bras were out, and showing cleavage in low-cut tops was in.

1980s   Big chests were back in fashion but on a slimmer form. Women headed to cosmetic surgeons for breast implants.

1990s   The Wonderbra appeared, promising cleavage to all. Women began coming forward with nightmare stories about their breast implants, leading to controversy over the safety of silicone implants.

2000s   Health concerns are shoved to the background and breast implants are back . . . and this time they've gone prime time with reality makeovers. We're manipulated to believe that perfect breasts are central to transforming an ugly duckling into a swan.

We have detached our breasts from their biological function and hoisted them into the realms of a fashion accessory.

-Jane Ogden, *Fat Chance!*

I must I must I must
I must increase my bust
The bigger the better
The tighter the sweater
I must increase my bust

–Exercise chant made popular in the 1950s

Breasts have gone far beyond their milk-making function. Breasts—boobs, tits, jugs, etcetera—can get even more attention than our personalities. Sometimes it seems as if they have personalities of their own, since they're commented on and stared at as if they were separate from us. Whether we develop early or late, are flat-chested, big-breasted, or somewhere in between, there is always some idiotic breast joke for our particular situation. Our own feelings about our breasts range from being happy about, proud of, or comfortable with them to wanting to stuff socks in our bras to boost them or wear baggy shirts to hide them. In 2003, more than 11,000 eighteen-year-olds had breast surgery—three times as many as the year before.[8] Ads offer "free breast implants" as a prize, but the risks are real: implants can ripple, rupture, cause nipple numbness and stretch marks, and interfere with breast-feeding—plus they need to be replaced every ten to twelve years.

Loving our breasts has nothing to do with their actual size, but with our confidence. The more comfortable we can be with our breasts, the less we'll care about others' opinions or how we "measure up."

Part of being comfortable with our breasts is being familiar with them and how they feel. The benefits of being well acquainted with our breasts are numerous. For one thing, 80 percent of breast cancer cases are found by self-exams. This does not necessarily mean we should only follow formal directions on how to conduct a breast self-exam. Feel your breasts however

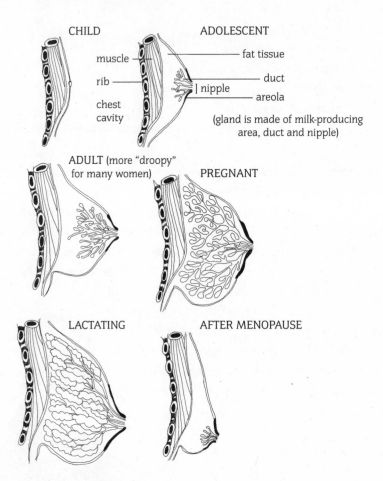

CHILD

ADOLESCENT

muscle

rib

chest
cavity

fat tissue

duct

| nipple

areola

(gland is made of milk-producing
area, duct and nipple)

ADULT (more "droopy"
for many women)

PREGNANT

LACTATING

AFTER MENOPAUSE

Breast changes over a lifetime.

and whenever you want to—it's important to get to know them so you can detect a change. And anyway, exploring and getting to know our bodies should not be like conducting a rigid regimen. We can be familiar with our breasts simply by holding them in our palms, massaging the skin with our fingers, and squeezing the nipples. Exploring our breasts should continue throughout our lives so that our fingers can sense any changes. Knowing our breasts also teaches us to be comfortable with our body as a whole. And, hey, touching our breasts is a pleasurable and affirming part of being female. So if you don't already, get to know them!

When exploring your breasts, you may notice some lumpiness. This is nothing to be alarmed about. Some women's breast tissue is fairly fine and feels smooth, while other women's tissue is very lumpy. Your breasts may be somewhere in between, with lumps near the armpits but smooth tissue below. During your period, your breasts go through changes, so the easiest time to notice any changes from the previous month is when your hormones are at their lowest (the last day of your period or right after). What you are looking for is anything that is out of the ordinary for *you*. Call your doctor if you have a concern, if you notice discharge from your nipples, or if the feel of your breasts seems different from your previous self-exam.

I kept waiting for mine to reach those stages.

In health class they would show us a chart of what your breasts are supposed to look like as they develop. So I kept waiting for mine to reach those stages. But my chest is flat and my breasts never looked like those charts. I felt cheated.

—Hennie, seventeen years old

I used to think my boobs were gigantic.

I was paranoid about it. I know they're my natural size, but it was hard because they just came on so quick. Over a short period of time I went from completely flat to the way I am now, which was hard to adjust to. I now wear the same bra size as my mother, which shocked me at first. I'm bigger than most of my friends, but now I'm comfortable with that.

—Reba, sixteen years old

I have a small chest, but it doesn't bother me.

I don't think guys care about chest size; they care if people are pretty. I knew a guy who was only going out with a friend of mine because she had a big chest. But I bet he personally didn't really care—he was just trying to impress his friends.

—China, fifteen years old

I have a friend whose mom got her breast implants for her eighteenth birthday.

That seems like an odd present to me, but my friend really wanted to be bustier. She gets more attention now, but she doesn't really seem any happier.

—Hannah, nineteen years old

Taking Back Our Bodies

Dissatisfaction with our bodies wastes time and can result in weight obsession. What difference would it make in your life if you suddenly had your ideal body? Would it really involve the changes you think? If we could be more accepting of our bodies, no matter what their size or shape, we would have more time and energy for creativity, friends, and who knows what else.

The practice of body acceptance is a courageous action, and one of the best things we can do for ourselves. How do we do this? We can be our own best resource and try some of the following practice:

- Avoid statements that put our bodies down, like "I hate my thighs/stomach/legs/ breasts . . ." We need to stop sending our bodies these negative signals, which only eat away at our self-esteem and honor. We can also point out negative self-talk among our friends and family, and support each other in transforming our words.

- Tell our bodies that we love them. We can create a daily practice (maybe in the shower or the bathtub as we scrub and lather each part) telling our bodies that we love, accept, and promise to take care of them as best we can. It's amazing what a little affection can do.

- Become media wise. We must educate ourselves by observing the types of images that are bombarding us from the magazines, movie screens, televisions, billboards, and catalogs. What are these images saying? How are they making us feel about ourselves? Our challenge is to accept our bodies as they are and to avoid making negative comparisons. If a magazine is making us feel consistently bad, we can cancel the subscription. And, while we're at it, we can write a letter to the editor explaining why we are canceling our subscription. Same thing with a TV show: Shutting it off can be a great political statement!

- Seek out alternative forms of media that honor and celebrate body diversity. If we usually read

Seventeen or *Glamour*, check out *Essence, Bust, Latina Style,* or *Radiance.* We can also read books or watch movies that depict cultures different than our own.

- Give up the fairy tale ending, "If we had the perfect body, then . . ." It is a sham and never leads to true happiness because there is always the next thing we need to "fix" or ways we can still "do better." The trick is to start having and doing all of the things we think we would do or have once we had that perfect body. It's funny how our bodies become perfect when we are fully engaged in doing what we love.

- Deal with our emotions instead of stuffing them. Sometimes we resort to dieting, binging, excessive exercising, or other unhealthy body behaviors as an attempt to deal with psychological or emotional issues. We are emotional beings, and we need to find healthy outlets for our feelings rather than transferring our anxieties about school, relationships, and life changes onto the shape and size of our bodies.

- Stand up for body acceptance by helping to combat the stereotypes and "sizisms" we live with. Have we or someone we know ever been discriminated against or hurt by comments made about body shape or size? How have we responded? How can we respond in a way that supports body acceptance?

I'm trying to open myself to other images of beauty.

I'm trying to redefine my definition of what makes a body beautiful. My old definition is a very thin, almost skeletal woman who doesn't have any curves whatsoever. Before, I was totally unaware that what I was thinking was hurting me. I think we need to reach a point where every body type is represented in the media and there is no one standard of beauty. We need to consider all body types as beautiful.

—Sandra, seventeen years old

3

Eating Disorders
When Eating Goes Way Out of Order

why do we crucify ourselves
every day I crucify myself
nothing I do is good enough for you
crucify myself every day
and my HEART is sick of being in chains
                    —Tori Amos, "Crucify," *Little Earthquakes*

We have an eating disorder when our eating is out of order. Anorexia nervosa and bulimia nervosa get the most media attention, but there are related disorders, such as compulsive overeating and binge eating. It's alarming but true: more than 90 percent of people with eating disorders are female adolescents.[1] The statistics are grim:

- About one out of every one hundred females suffers from anorexia.[2]

- About two to three out of every one hundred females will develop bulimia nervosa.[3]

- Up to fifteen out of one hundred people report eating behaviors that are disturbed: vomiting after meals, feeling out of control when eating, or restricting food intake to an obsessive level.[4]

- About half of the individuals with anorexia or bulimia have a full recovery, while 30 percent have a partial recovery and 20 percent have no substantial improvement.[5]

Why are these disorders overwhelmingly female, and why do so many of us have them? There is no clear answer, but from the age of seven, girls begin showing more concern than boys do about body weight and shape. And this difference in attitudes only increases with age. Growing up, boys don't seem to face the same anxiety about feeling too big or taking up too much space.

I was normal, but I felt huge compared to everyone else.

My effort to lose weight began when I was ten. I was already five feet, four inches tall, and that's big for that age. All the other girls were very thin and small, petite. I was normal, but I felt huge compared to everyone else. I started eating just one real meal a day. I had no time for breakfast in the morning, and for lunch I would maybe have a slice of bread. At night I would have a no-fat, no-salt dinner. I was basically starving. I definitely wanted to lose weight and be thin and beautiful, but I got so skinny it was scary. I got down to ninety pounds, and at the time, I still didn't feel thin. Now, I see pictures of myself, and I looked awful: My hair was in horrible shape, it was frizzy and brittle; my teeth were terrible; my skin was in bad shape; and I had dark circles under my eyes. I did not look healthy. I got over it in the sixth grade, when I moved back in with my dad, who is super supportive and an amazing cook.

—Margo, sixteen years old

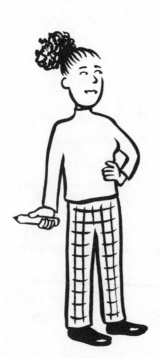
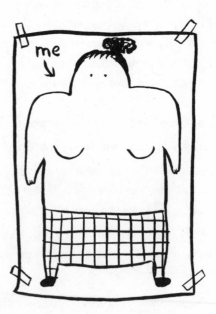

Swallow

Where are all the girls who withered
inside the cornucopia?
a pile of deflowered bodies,
gray bones and crystal teeth
shattered among the breakfast dishes.
Like a cold pasta dream,
they've been left beneath the eyelids
where colors are calories
and shapes only
fragments of the meals.
Lifting the hand to mouth,
I spy the pockets of rolling flesh,
I breathe the crushing nourishment
and quietly swallow the scale.

—Robin, seventeen years old

An Emotional Hunger? A Need for Control?

Why does one girl spend her high school years focusing on her weight and struggling with binging and purging, while another goes through her teen years unfazed by how much she eats and weighs? There's no one answer to why young girls develop eating disorders, why we gravitate—almost like flies to flypaper—to food and weight as our focus for obsessive behavior. Individual personalities, family attitudes, cultural traditions, and media influences may be important factors. And if we belong to a group that places an importance on thinness, such as ballet dancers, gymnasts, models, long-distance runners, or other body-conscious teens, we may find ourselves surrounded by an eating-disorder culture. Some girls find that the attention they get when they start to lose weight is the start of a seductive, vicious cycle.

There are certainly many theories out there about the causes of eating disorders, and it can be overwhelming to sort through them in all the self-help books that are available these days, such as *Feeding the Hungry Heart, When Food Is Love,* or *You Can't Quit 'til You Know What's Eating You.* The following list offers some theories about why we turn food into a weapon against ourselves. There is no one right answer—the answer for each person may be a unique combination of social, biological, psychological, and familial issues. We should pick and choose whatever hits home.

- We use fatness or skinniness as a shield, or to hide from others.
- We escape difficult emotions (fear, sadness, anxiety, anger) by overeating, starving, binging, or purging.
- We turn a simple diet or unintentional weight loss into an unhealthy fixation.
- We have a biological makeup that makes us more likely to develop an addictive behavior.
- We are part of a social or athletic environment that demands thinness for success.
- We have a mother or father who is critical of our appearance.
- We are in conflict with or seek approval from a parent.
- We rebel against the pressure to diet by overeating or extreme dieting.
- We diet because we fear growing up or being independent.
- The media projects the "ideal" woman as someone twenty pounds under-weight, making us feel fat and therefore undesirable.
- We want to take up as little space as possible and not be a threat to anyone.
- We avoid dealing with our sexuality by burying ourselves in thoughts about food.
- So much of life is out of our control, and food intake is one of the things we can control.
- We want attention.
- We live in a society that objectifies women and encourages us to fixate on our bodies.
- We substitute an obsession with food and weight for personal relationships.
- We don't feel good enough or accepted and loved for who we are.
- We have a history of familial abuse or sexual abuse.

The Hungry Self

These books offer insight and support to those of us struggling with food issues:

The Body Betrayed: A Deeper Understanding of Women, Eating Disorders, and Treatment by Kathryn J. Zerbe, Carlsbad, CA: Gürze Books, 1995.

Breaking Free from Emotional Eating by Geneen Roth, New York: Plume Books, 2003.

Eating in the Light of the Moon: How Women Can Transform Their Relationships with Food through Myths, Metaphors, and Storytelling by Anita Johnston, Carlsbad, CA: Gürze Books, 2000.

Fed Up!: The Breakthrough Ten-Step, No-Diet Fitness Plan by Wendy Oliver-Pyatt, New York: McGraw Hill, 2004.

Good Enough . . . When Losing Is Winning, and Thin Enough Can Never Be Achieved by Cynthia Bitter, Penfield, NY: Hopelines, 1998.

Hunger Pains: The Modern Woman's Tragic Quest for Thinness by Mary Pipher, New York: Ballantine Books, 1997.

A Hunger So Wide and So Deep: American Women Speak Out on Eating Problems by Becky W. Thompson, Minneapolis: University of Minnesota Press, 1996.

The Hungry Self: Women, Eating, and Identity by Kim Chernin, New York: Perennial Books, 1994.

Inner Hunger by Marianne Apostolides, New York: W. W. Norton, 1998.

Perk! The Story of a Teenager with Bulimia by Liza F. Hall, Carlsbad, CA: Gürze Books, 1997.

The Secret Language of Eating Disorders: How You Can Understand and Work to Cure Anorexia and Bulimia by Peggy Claude-Pierre, New York: Vintage, 1998.

What Are You Hungry For?: Women, Food, and Spirituality by Lynn Ginsburg and Mary Taylor, New York: St. Martin's, 2002.

The pressure to be thin is all over.

I think there are so many eating disorders because the pressure to be thin is all over, in the media and in our peer groups. When you are young, you are trying to decide how you want to be and how you want to look. When you see ads or movies where men only look at skinny women, you think that is the only way you are going to get attention or get complimented.

—Sheri, eighteen years old

Her mom told her she couldn't get any new clothes until she lost ten pounds.

I hate when moms tell daughters to watch what they eat. I had a friend who was always a normal weight. In eighth grade, her mom told her she couldn't get any new clothes for the next season until she lost ten pounds. But she didn't need to lose any weight. She ended up losing way over that and became really sick. She was anorexic. She exercised all the time and took that to an extreme. No one could understand why her mother, who is a nurse, couldn't see what her daughter was doing. My mom always worries that I'm not eating enough, even when I have tons. My mom always wants to feed people, so it was weird to me that her mom was putting pressure on her to lose weight.

—Rose, eighteen years old

Dieting for me was an attempt to get my old self back.

Before puberty, I was stick thin and never thought about my body or what I ate. Then, almost overnight, I grew boobs and hips and I felt completely awkward. I would walk around with my books in front of my chest and wear baggy, baggy clothes. Losing weight for me was an attempt to get my old self back. I gave up on dieting when I joined the field hockey team and realized that my strength was more important. I'm now comfortable with my size, but it took some adjustment.

—Maggie, fifteen years old

A lot of people blame the media . . . I think that is just an excuse.

A lot of people blame the media for anorexia and bulimia, but I think that is just an excuse; they use the media as a scapegoat. The problem is a lot of girls want to look like the models, but there is variation in human beings. There's not a super-model mold.

—Becca, eighteen years old

Why are magazines trying to put that image across?

I blame the fashion industry for causing eating disorders. Why can't they put clothes on a person with a normal body? I hate super skinny models. I don't even think people are attractive when they look too skinny. Yet this is the image young girls think they have to look like. Maybe you could look like that if you starved yourself. But why would you want to? I think it's a really bad image to give off to teenage girls. The majority of people don't have bodies like that.

The media could change things. If we had more models of all different body shapes, that would help girls calm down. What's wrong with being average?

—Margot, sixteen years old

Compulsive Overeating: Emotional Stuffing

It's possible to feel that our eating is out of control no matter what our size or shape. We regularly feel as if we can't stop eating, and our lack of control makes us feel terrible and guilty. We struggle to stop, but find ourselves flipping between overeating and making strict promises about our eating habits that are impossible to maintain. As compulsive overeaters, many of us place a lot of importance on and have an intense anxiety about our body shape and weight. We also tend to have unrealistic diet standards and a preoccupation with food. These concerns are similar to those of people with other eating disorders.

As compulsive overeaters, we may be using food as a way to deal with emotional upset. Food can be a companion, a comfort, and an escape. Children are often given food treats as a reward, so certain foods carry memories of approval or security. Most of us, at one time or another, turn to food when we are unhappy, worried, angry, or excited. But if we are compulsive overeaters, we tend to be food-focused. We often eat according to our emotions, and our overeating tends to be secretive and out of control. Instead of dealing with difficult feelings, we numb out with food. If

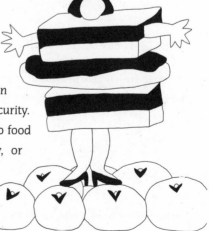

"I just ate a box tangerines, three cakes, and three pastries and now this is how I feel."

overeating leads to obesity, the fatness can be a way to protect ourselves from other people. For example, we may avoid hanging out with friends because we feel unattractive.

Talking about the feelings that lead to overeating with friends or with an adult we trust may help us stop both the pattern of emotional stuffing and the overeating. There are also support groups, such as Overeaters Anonymous, that provide a place for individuals with similar issues to come together and work on getting beyond the compulsion to overeat. Check out the sidebar on the page 69 for a list of books that provide an in-depth look at eating issues.

I finally realized I would need an entire shelf of cookies to drown out all the confused feelings I had.

When my mom told me to slim down, I just gained more weight. I don't get along with my mother, and I was against whatever she did. I ate bags of potato chips and pints of ice cream and felt like I couldn't stop. In secret, I would eat everything out of the fridge until I felt sick and bloated. After a binge, I'd wonder what was wrong with me and go to sleep miserable and puffy. I finally realized I would need an entire shelf of cookies to drown out all the confused feelings I had.

This year I talked to a therapist because of family problems. I figured out that I eat a lot when I am depressed or mad. I realized it is better to try to understand my actual feelings instead of trying to bury them in food.

—Nona, sixteen years old

Anorexia Nervosa: A Slow Road to Self-Destruction

According to the clinical definition of anorexia, a girl with anorexia nervosa has the following symptoms. Some of us may not show all of these symptoms but may still be in danger.

1. She has an intense fear of gaining weight or getting fat even though she is underweight.

2. She is less than 85 percent of her expected healthy weight and refuses to keep her weight within a normal weight range for her age and height.

3. She has a disturbed body image: She feels fat even when she is well below her ideal body weight; she denies the seriousness of her current low body weight; and her body shape or weight has extreme influence on her self-image.

4. She has amenorrhea—absence of menstruation—and has missed her period for at least the past three months, or is only able to get her period with the help of hormones such as estrogen.

There are two types of anorexia nervosa:

- The **bulimic anorexic** has symptoms 1–4 listed on the previous page and regularly engages in binging and purging behaviors (see description of bulimia nervosa in the next section).
- The **restrictive anorexic** has symptoms 1–4 but does not engage in the binging and purging behavior that characterizes bulimia nervosa.

Some of us may be envious of the willpower of an anorexic who successfully loses weight. But in reality, anorexia is ugly. As anorexics, we often feel miserable, alone, and cut off from the rest of the world. Our obsession with weight and food becomes the main focus of our lives.

Food was almost all I thought about during my four years of high school. It was a tragic waste of my time and energy.

In eighth grade, my friend gave me a calorie-counter book and I decided to go on a diet. When I get into things, I really get into things. I went away to camp thinking, "Calories—wow!" Now I had a new focus for my life. I figured, if I ate 1,500 calories a day and lost weight gradually, why not eat 300 a day, lose weight quickly, and get it over with? It was a big challenge to me. I felt good when I was hungry because it meant that it was working. I also started running to lose more weight. I came back from camp ten pounds lighter. It's weird, because I went to camp a normal person, and I came home not normal at all. All in the span of five weeks.

Back at school, everyone was into diets in one way or another. We were only thirteen years old. People gave me attention because I was thinner. I started taking diet pills and obsessing more and more. Some girls were public about their dieting and even formed friendships based on losing weight, but I was more secretive. I used to go to the mall every day and try on jeans as a way of escaping and gauging my weight. There was also a scale at the mall, and I'd weigh myself. The whole time I was dieting I felt like I was gaining weight. I saw myself as a little overweight and was afraid I would gain more.

I started to read about anorexics because I wanted to succeed at losing weight. My dad is a doctor, and I would read his casebooks. I was fascinated by their stories and wanted to pick up new techniques. I didn't think of myself as an anorexic because I thought you had to weigh like eighty pounds. I thought I was a "wanna-be."

Food was almost all I thought about during my four years of high school. It was a tragic waste of my time and energy. Worrying if I was eating too much and running enough was a huge endeavor. I was always thinking about food, planning everything out, and feeling bad about it. I can't even imagine high school without my eating disorder. I used it in an entirely escapist way, which everyone seems to. I thought if I was "this much" thinner then everything would be okay. My moods revolved around food. If everything was crazy and somebody didn't like me, I would think, "I'm losing weight, so everything is fine," or "I'm gaining weight, so everything sucks." On one hand it's about how your body looks, and on the other it has nothing to do with your body. It felt like something mentally addictive. Once it gets into your head, it's like cancer spreading from one place to another. Anorexia ended up taking more control of my life than I took control of it.

I finally improved by realizing I had a problem. I talked with a friend of mine who had the same experiences. It helped me realize I wasn't the only one and I wasn't crazy. I started putting myself into books, like The Best Little Girl in the World, *as someone who had the problem, not someone who was aspiring to have the problem. It all got old. I wondered how I'd feel looking back on my life: "Do I want to think I spent 90 percent of my life just trying to be a certain weight?" I started getting into feminism too and realized worrying about weight is oppressive.*

Now I'm the weight I think I should be; back then I was ninety-eight pounds. I eat almost anything I want now, and I never count calories.

—Monica, seventeen years old

I was constantly cold and sick all the time. There were definite signs that should have alerted me that something was the matter.

I'm not sure how my anorexia began; it evolved over a year. In eighth grade it was a trend for girls to be on a diet. I started out on a diet, and it got worse from there. First I was slightly restricting my calories; then I was eating just salad. I started to calculate calories, writing calories down and seeing how much I could reduce them each week. By the summer before ninth grade I was pretty sick.

I stopped getting my period for over a year, but I didn't think that was serious. I just thought, "Oh, this must mean I'm doing really well with my dieting." I was constantly cold and sick all the time. There were definite signs that should have alerted me that something was the matter, but I thought they were signs that I was definitely losing weight and that "I'm doing well with this." If I wasn't feeling sick, I felt something was wrong. My mind put everything in total reverse.

I didn't see myself as overweight, but I never saw myself as thin, either. I saw myself as the same size that I was before I started losing weight. Even when I

Eating Disorders in History

Myth: Anorexia nervosa and bulimia nervosa are new disorders and just fads.

Reality: Anorexia nervosa and bulimia nervosa were defined over one hundred years ago. Similar symptoms have been described for hundreds of years.

Eating disorder symptoms are nothing new. Here are some examples from centuries ago:

☀ Friderade was a serf who lived in the ninth century. Soon after recovering from an illness, she mysteriously developed a mammoth appetite and took to gorging herself on food. Like many modern-day bulimics, Friderade felt ashamed about her behavior. As a way of battling her eating habits, which disgusted her, she went to a monastery, where she began restricting her food intake. As she fasted, she became extremely thin but continued to work long hours despite her weakening condition. Friderade's story is similar to modern-day cases of anorexia nervosa (bulimic type) in many ways: She had cycles of overeating followed by fasting; she was secretive and felt guilty about her eating habits; she refused to think she needed help, denying that anything was wrong with her; and she continued to be physically active despite being dangerously thin.[1]

☀ In the thirteenth century, "holy" women starved themselves to become more acceptable in God's eyes. Their starvation was only one form of their self-denial; others included sleeping on boards, hitting themselves with iron chains, wearing scratchy woolen clothing, and praying for hours on end in a kneeling position. Though these women gave religious reasons for their starvation, it's likely that some suffered from anorexia nervosa.

☀ The term "bulimia nervosa" was first used in 1873, and bulimia's literal meaning is "appetite like an ox." The term "anorexia nervosa" was first used in 1874, and anorexia literally means "loss of appetite or desire." Bulimia was not considered to be a separate disorder from anorexia until 1980.[2]

☀ In 1994, binge eating disorder was added to the DSM IV, the fourth edition of the Diagnostic Manual of Mental Disorders, as a distinct type of eating disorder.

reached ninety pounds, I still looked the same way in the mirror. When my parents or others said I was losing weight, I took it as a twisted compliment. After I was getting psychological and medical treatment and starting to gain the weight back, the hardest thing for me to deal with was the loss of attention. People were no longer telling me, "You're sooo skinny!" or "You're too skinny; you look like you need to gain weight." I was just normal again.

—Polly, seventeen years old

Bulimia Nervosa: It's a Vicious Cycle

Bulimia nervosa is a more common eating disorder than anorexia nervosa. Studies show that two to three out of every one hundred adolescent and young adult women suffer from bulimia; however, this number may be even higher since bulimics have a tendency to be secretive about their disorder.[6]

According to the clinical definition of bulimia, a girl with bulimia nervosa has the following symptoms. Some of us may not show these exact symptoms but may still need help:

1. She is overconcerned with her body shape and weight.
2. She binges at least two times per week. *Binging* is consuming a large quantity of food in a short period of time (usually within a two-hour time span) and feeling out of control while consuming the food. The food that is eaten during a binge is often sweet and easily swallowed, like ice cream or cake, or salty, like potato chips, or high in carbohydrates, like pasta. A binge may be planned or unplanned and is generally done in private and kept secret from others.
3. Her binging is regularly followed by purging. *Purging* is any activity that gets rid of or counteracts the food consumed during the binge: self-induced vomiting, taking laxatives or enemas (to speed up bowel movements), taking diuretics (to make you urinate), fasting, or exercising excessively.

There are two types of bulimia nervosa:

- **Purging type:** The individual regularly engages in self-induced vomiting or misuses laxatives, enemas, or diuretics.
- **Non-purging type:** Though this is called "non-purging," the individual actually is purging by fasting or through excessive exercise, and does not regularly engage in self-induced vomiting or the misuse of laxatives or diuretics.

A bulimic (who is not a "bulimic anorexic"; see description of anorexia nervosa types) is usually of normal body weight (within ten to fifteen pounds of her ideal weight range) and differs from an anorexic in the following ways:[7]

1. Though she is very concerned with her weight and appearance, a bulimic has a more realistic perception of her body than an anorexic does.
2. She is more likely to acknowledge her abnormal eating patterns.
3. She is more impulsive—suddenly acting on something without thinking about it or the consequences ahead of time.
4. She is more likely to seek out and get treatment for her eating disorder, and her recovery time is usually shorter.

Bulimics describe binges as having a numbing effect on emotions. For example, if we are bulimic and feel angry or anxious, we try to get rid of or stuff down the emotion by binging on food. The binge, however, makes us feel guilty, and we often describe hating ourselves. The purging is used to get rid of our self-hatred and guilt, by actually getting rid of the food consumed during the binge. The purging provides us with both physical and emotional relief, but also adds to the distress of the whole behavior. We wonder, "How can I keep doing this to myself?" In the end, we feel as angry or anxious as we did before the cycle began.

Somewhere in me I had always known it wasn't natural to throw up everything I ate.

My bulimia started in tenth grade. I compared my eating to others and felt guilty for eating more. It's kind of funny, but I always aspired to be anorexic. I'd say, "Okay, I'm just not going to eat tomorrow," but I would eat. When I had eaten what I thought was too much, I would feel nauseated and guilty. It occurred to me, "You've eaten too much, and you should do something about it." I started by throwing up one meal a day. Then it got to the point where I would throw up many times each day, even a couple of times during one meal.

I don't think people at school knew about my bulimia. During dinner, I would often go into the basement bathroom. Other times, I would walk out into the woods that were behind the dorms to throw up. I kept it a secret from my family, too.

Throwing up affected my whole mind-set. Whenever I ate, afterwards there was only one thought in my mind, "Where can I go to throw up?" It strained my friendships. If I was with someone and I ate something, I'd be trying to talk to them and be my "normal" self, but at the same time my mind was racing. I was trying to figure out when I could get away for long enough to throw up. It was terrible. I couldn't focus on anything else; I couldn't forget it.

Sometimes I would make a vow, like, "I'll go to breakfast and only eat half a grapefruit and a bowl of cereal." Occasionally it would work, but usually I'd eat more than that, feel bad, and throw up. It was a cycle that was self-created. I would set a limit for how much I should eat, and if I went over it then it was all gone: "Since I've gone over, I'm going to have to throw up, so I might as well eat anything I want." In the end I ate more than normal since I decided I was a failure anyway. I wanted to lose weight, but I stayed the same weight. I knew I had bulimia, but I felt disconnected from it. I knew all the terrible things that could happen to me. I would read, "Sometimes bulimics die because their electrolytes become imbalanced and they have a heart attack." I thought, "That's not me in the story, so it's all right."

Months after I started, it seemed to be getting easier to throw up. After a meal I would naturally start gagging. At that point I realized, "If my body is naturally doing this, then that's how it's supposed to be." This continued almost all of my sophomore year. Then I don't know exactly what changed, but all of a sudden I was scared. I was scared that my body was being so weird. I became less capable of eating something and not throwing up. I decided it had to stop. Too much of my time was consumed by throwing up, and so many of my thoughts were centered on it. My hands were all scratched up from gagging. Of course somewhere in me I had always known that it wasn't natural to throw up everything I ate. But I became worried that I would never be able to eat something and not throw up. I was also feeling more isolated because I was spending less time with my friends. I felt that I had to excuse myself often and felt awkward, so I spent less time with them. I decided to go to the school counselor and deal with what I was doing to myself.

—Lisa, seventeen years old

It's hard to talk to someone about their eating disorder, but I feel it's important to try.

These days I'm over the worst of my bulimia, but I still have days where I binge and then want to purge. I now know that it has a lot to do with my stress level. If I'm stressed and eat three bowls of cereal, then I will want to get rid of it, even though rationally I know that three bowls of cereal isn't worth throwing up over. In the past, I could not have distinguished that it was related to how I was feeling.

I definitely think there is something contagious about eating disorders. This spring, my entire class went to a pizza parlor. A friend went to the bathroom, and she said that every stall was filled with someone throwing up. It's hard to talk to someone else about their eating disorder, but I feel it's important to try. I always come from the support side. I told someone in my class: "I heard you throwing up; I used to do that all the time. I can't say I know how you are feeling, but I think I have a good idea, and if you ever want to talk about it, I'm always here."

My turning point was when I finally talked to others about my bulimia. It was during summer camp after the tenth grade and I told my closest friend, "You were right, I was throwing up because I'm bulimic." That was important because it wasn't a secret anymore—my whole cabin knew and was supportive. It really helped to talk about it.

—Elizabeth, seventeen years old

Binge Eating Disorder

Binge eating disorder has only recently been defined by the medical community. As many as four out of every one hundred adolescent and young women suffer from binge eating—making it the most common eating disorder.[8]

Like bulimics, if we are binge eaters we have recurrent binges which are characterized by: a large amount of food that is consumed in a short period of time (within two hours), a strong feeling of being out of control over what is being eaten, and a sense of not being able to stop. For a girl with binge eating disorder, binges take place, on average, at least two days per week (and may be as often as multiple times in one day), cause marked distress, and are associated with three or more of the following symptoms:

1. She eats much more rapidly than she normally would.
2. She eats until she feels uncomfortable.
3. She eats large amounts of food when not feeling physically hungry.
4. She eats alone because she is embarrassed by how much she is eating.
5. She feels disgusted with herself, depressed, or very guilty after overeating.

Unlike bulimics, if we have binge eating disorder, we do not purge. Binge eating disorder is often overlooked by healthcare providers because it is not as well known as anorexia and bulimia, and the binging is often misclassified as simply a lack of discipline or a "fat person" problem. If we have binge eating disorder, we are most likely overweight, but people of average weight are also affected. Those of us who are obese and have binge eating disorder often become overweight at a younger age than those without the disorder. As binge eaters, we often suffer from the yo-yo diet syndrome, where we lose and gain back weight over and over.[9]

The causes of binge eating are still unknown, but up to half of us with the disorder have also experienced depression, and many of us report that anger, sadness, boredom, anxiety, or other negative emotions trigger these binges. It has also been found that strict dieting may worsen the disorder, as the restricting simply sets us up for our next binge.[10]

As we gain more clarity and understanding about binge eating disorder, as well as compulsive overeating, anorexia, and bulimia, we become better at educating and supporting others about these issues, and at establishing the most effective recovery techniques.

Binging

I am eating in overdrive, everything tastes of cheese.
I feel huge and porous as a water-slug. The kitchen

is in black and white, I'm in black and white.
Only the food is alive: Cheeto-orange, vibrating,

electric. It glows inside me like a barium test.
You could power a TV with this energy, you could feed

a thousand starving kids, hell, you could run
the whole city of Pittsburgh off these quivering

shrink-wrapped brownies and Twizzlers, candy bars
and potato chips. I want that energy. I want to consume

until I find infinity in these pulsing blocks of food, until
I am a network of colors branching out like bronchial tubes.

It does not end, this search. I can barely chew anymore.
My throat is scorched with vomit. But I can't stop looking,

can't stop flinging kitchen cabinets open, tearing
through plastic bags with my teeth, waiting to be consumed.

–Robin, seventeen years old

Not Quite Anorexia or Bulimia: Undefined Suffering

We can suffer from disordered eating but not fit the full description of either anorexia nervosa, bulimia nervosa, or binge eating disorder; this is sometimes referred to as "an eating disorder not otherwise specified." For example, we can feel obsessed with losing weight and worrying about what we eat but never lose an amount of weight that puts our health in jeopardy, or we can have all of the symptoms of anorexia but never lose our period. We may make ourselves throw up after only small amounts of food (like two cookies); or we may binge and feel extremely guilty about the binging but never do it frequently enough to be diagnosed with a disorder. Eating is disordered when it gets in the way of our life: We don't go out because we feel too fat; we can't eat around other people; we spend an enormous amount of time thinking or worrying about food. Whether or not we fit into a classic definition of anorexia, bulimia, or binge eating disorder, suffering is suffering, there are potentially life-threatening results, and it's important to seek help (see section "What If I Have an Eating Disorder? Get Help!").

No one with an eating disorder is alone, even though you feel totally alone.

Everyone I've talked to started their eating disorders in similar ways, whether it's bulimia, anorexia, a mixture of both, or not quite either. This shows that no one with an eating disorder is alone, even though you feel totally alone. There are many girls who not only feel the same way about their weight but who have the same patterns of eating and obsession.

—Leila, seventeen years old

I wish I had known that not getting my period was something that was really bad for me.

Anorexia is not a cool thing. I think an important thing to focus on is how dangerous it is on an emotional level, and a physical level. I wish I had known that not getting my period was something that was really bad for me. When somebody is in the midst of an eating disorder, it's hard to make an emotional appeal and tell them, "You're hurting yourself." I think it's much better to make a logical appeal and present the facts: You're going to get sick, and it's going to be really hard to recover.

—Sarah, seventeen years old

Knowing Someone with an Eating Disorder

Chances are we know someone who has struggled with an eating disorder or is in the middle of dealing with one. Eating disorders are stressful on friendships, especially given the likelihood of an anorexic girl to deny any problem and the tendency toward secrecy among girls with bulimia and binge eating disorder. An eating disorder is not contagious, of course, but it takes perspective to stay relaxed about weight and food issues when others around us are not. We can support friends with eating disorders by letting them know we are concerned and recommending that they seek professional help. The following is a helpful list of tips from the Harvard Eating Disorders Center (www.hedc.org) for approaching and speaking to a friend who is struggling with an eating disorder.

Before approaching your friend:
- Find out about resources for help in your community so that you can offer her a strategy to connect with that help (see the sidebar "Getting Help for Eating Problems" on pages 90–91).
- Consider getting advice and support from someone, like a counselor at school, about the situation.
- Increase your own understanding by reading about eating disorders (read this chapter and see the sidebar on page 69 for some additional resources).
- Plan ahead to make enough time to talk to your friend without being interrupted.
- Choose a cozy, safe, and private place to talk.

Ideas for what to say:
- Begin by telling your friend how much you care about her.
- Next, offer some reflections about her emotional state, such as: "You seem unhappy/preoccupied/anxious/fidgety/distant/jumpy/angry, and I'm worried about you."
- Give your friend a few observations about her behavior to explain why you think she might have an eating disorder. For example: "I see you skip meals/I watch you run to the bathroom/I hear you talk all the time about being afraid of being fat, what you ate, how much you're going to exercise, etc."
- If she tells you that she doesn't have a problem, or that she can stop on her own, you can say something like, "Eating disorders can be like addictions,

where it is hard to see you have a serious problem and that you need help. I hear what you're saying, but I think you're really struggling and you need help stopping. I believe in you, and I know you deserve to get help and get better."

- If she refuses to get help, tell her that you are not going to bug her, but that you are also not going to stop being concerned either. For example: "Even if I can't convince you to get help now, I can't stop caring."

Dos and Don'ts:
- Do speak from your heart, using "I" statements.
- Don't get into a "Yes, you do/No, I don't" argument.
- Do stay calm, even if your friend gets upset or angry.
- Don't name other people who are also worried about her because that can feel like you are ganging up on her.
- Do remind her that friends tell friends when they are worried about them.
- Don't take all the responsibility for your friend's problems on your shoulders alone—tell a teacher, a counselor, or your friend's mother or father that you are concerned.
- Do give your friend information about who can help her, and offer to go with her.

It may take more than one approach before she will agree to get help. And your friend may continue to refuse to get help. We must realize that she needs to take the step toward recovery herself and that we cannot make her do anything.

If your friend is getting help for her eating disorder:
- Stay connected to her the same way you would with any friend (call her, invite her to do things, hang out, and ask her for advice about your life).
- When talking with her about herself, do not focus on her eating disorder (most people with eating disorders feel embarrassed about them and feel safer in friendships in which friends do not try to get involved in the details of the disorder).
- Avoid all comments—even compliments—about looks, weight, food intake, or clothes (including about her, you, and other people).
- Avoid giving her advice on how she could change her behavior.
- Do not ask a lot of questions about her recovery.
- Remember that recovery takes time.

I finally decided to call her mom and tell her what was going on.
    One of my good friends, Marta, started starving herself. Marta is a smart and good person, so it really bothered me. I told her she was being stupid. She knew when other people had eating disorders, but couldn't see it for herself. I said, "It's scary, you don't see you are among those people." She replied, "How can you accuse me of that?" In one day she only eats plain pasta or a bagel. After she finishes her bagel, she complains, "I feel so fat." Marta is weight crazy. One night, we had plans for the evening. She used to make me lie to her mom and say that she had been eating with me. I finally decided to call her mom and tell her what was going on. Her mom said, "Are you sure? She said she was eating with you." She told me she would poke around. I told her not to say anything to Marta, and she didn't. I left it up to her mom to deal with her eating issues, and I stayed friends with Marta.
    —Blossom, eighteen years old

What If I Have an Eating Disorder? Get Help!

Some of us with mild eating disorders are able to recover by ourselves or by sharing our secretive behavior with a supportive friend, but a lot of us find that seeking professional help is a major factor in healing and recovery. To get started, we can: talk with a school counselor or our family physician; contact our local hospital and inquire about eating disorder programs and services; get in touch with the student health services at a local college (which often have eating disorder programs); call the Eating Disorders Awareness and Prevention hotline at (800) 931-2237; or ask a local counseling center for a referral to an eating disorders specialist or self-help group.

    We may find it hard to seek help for many reasons—shame, guilt, fear, hopelessness, denial, or simply because we think we can or should be able to handle our problems ourselves. However, it can be a huge relief to share our concerns with someone else. Most of us have to first let go of our concerns about weight and eating before we can start to get better. And understanding why we have an eating disorder is usually the key to recovering and remaining healthy.

    It can take years for some of us to fully get over an eating disorder. In severe cases, anorexics and bulimics may need to be hospitalized. Recovery is a process, and setbacks can happen. Sometimes after recovering, we fall back into an eating disorder or go from one type to another, most commonly from anorexia to bulimia. Successful treatment for eating disorders often consists of several layers of support, including counseling, group or family therapy, nutritional counseling, and/or prescribed medications, such as antidepressants. It's important that we find the treatment that best fits our needs. Talking to a professional counselor or therapist may help us understand what is going on in our life that makes us turn to—or away from—food in a destructive way, and help us get on the road to recovery.

I didn't see that I was anorexic.

I didn't recognize I had a problem to deal with. My parents finally took me to a doctor and a psychiatrist, but it took a while for their counseling to sink in. In the beginning I told the doctor, "This isn't helping me at all." I didn't see that I was anorexic. I began taking medication for depression, which alleviated a lot of my symptoms. It made me think that some of my problem was biochemical. Drugs didn't erase the problem, but they helped me. Seeing my psychiatrist was what got me to the root of my problems, although in the beginning I wouldn't have admitted that. I would have been much worse off if I hadn't gone to a psychiatrist.

—Polly, seventeen years old

Taking away the secretiveness made it carry less importance for me.

I finally admitted that I was bulimic to my close friend. That was important because she was supportive. Taking away the secretiveness made it carry less importance for me. She told me, "I know you are doing this, and I don't think it's good, but I still like you." It helped to know someone who knew about my bulimia and still accepted me.

I talked to the school counselor, who helped me see how I used throwing up as an emotional relief. Binging and throwing up was a symbolic way of getting rid of my stress. I used throwing up like a drug. I don't know how I had the willpower, but I started to throw up less. I would have to rationalize not throwing up: "It's been an hour since I ate, so there is no point in throwing up now." The counselor helped me to stop, but it's still hard. I threw up once a few months ago, and about twice a year I have the urge. Those times, after I eat and feel full, I get a nagging voice that says, "Maybe you should get rid of that food." I've learned that stress triggers my wanting to throw up. The more responsibilities I have, the more I'm likely to hear that voice. Now I have a talk with that voice and tell it how I don't really want to throw up, but I want to get rid of the stress that I'm under. I'll say to myself, "You shouldn't throw up because that won't get rid of any of the stress. What you need to do is figure out why you're under so much stress and do something about it." Then I'll go and listen to music, clean my room, or talk to a friend.

—Claudia, seventeen years old

Having an Eating Disorder: It Ain't Pretty

Eating disorders are not glamorous. Anorexia and bulimia nervosa are both physically and emotionally damaging; if not treated, they can lead to permanent health complications and, in some rare cases, death. The following is a list of potential consequences from anorexia, bulimia, compulsive overeating, and binge eating disorder:[1]

Social Consequences of an Eating Disorder

- Relationships with family and friends become dysfunctional, manipulative, or nonexistent
- Social activity diminishes or stops altogether

Mental and Emotional Consequences of an Eating Disorder

- Obsessive thoughts
- Difficulty concentrating and thinking
- Depression

Physical Complications of Anorexia Nervosa

- Development of fine body hair (called lanugo) from severe weight loss
- Hypothermia (low body temperature)
- Lowered blood pressure
- Slowed pulse rate
- Slow heart rate or disturbances in the heart's rhythm
- Fatigue and lack of energy
- Dizziness and headaches
- Insomnia
- Imbalances in body chemistry from vitamin and nutrient deficiencies (also known as electrolyte imbalances)
- Low white blood cell count
- Stunted growth
- Osteoporosis (loss of bone mass, so that bones get brittle and break easily)
- Bloating
- Constipation
- Amenorrhea (absence of menstruation)
- Physiological dependence on the "high" produced by endorphins (a morphine-like substance produced by a body under stress)

- Damage to pancreas, kidneys, and even the heart and brain if malnutrition continues
- Skin problems
- Hair loss and nail damage
- Infertility

Physical Complications of Bulimia Nervosa

Binging:

- Hypoglycemia, a sugar deficiency leading to dizziness, headaches, fatigue, irritability, numbness, anxiety, and depression
- Lethargy, inactivity, lowered metabolism
- Headaches and dizziness

Purging:

- Erosion of tooth enamel from vomiting
- Bleeding in the esophagus
- Mouth sores and gum disease
- Edema (swelling caused by the accumulation of watery fluid in the tissues or cavities of the body)
- Imbalances in body chemistry from vitamin and nutrient deficiencies
- Dehydration

- Loss of skin elasticity
- Low blood pressure
- Heart irregularities
- Gastric dilation (enlargement of stomach and related areas)
- Constipation and bowel problems from overuse of laxatives
- Seizures

Physical Complications of Compulsive Overeating

- Weight gain
- Fatigue
- Heart irregularities
- Diabetes
- Varicose veins
- High blood pressure
- Shortness of breath
- High cholesterol levels

Physical Complications of Binge Eating Disorder

- High blood pressure and cholesterol
- Kidney disease and/or failure
- Arthritis
- Bone deterioration
- Heart attack
- Stroke

What We Miss When We Have an Eating Disorder: Life

I definitely have more time than I did when I was sick.

My bulimia was a weight I carried around like a secret, a big hunk of lead that I always had in my pocket. I wouldn't go out with a friend if I knew it was going to be hard to get to a bathroom. I could have been doing so many other things: going out with my friends, reading, writing, listening to music, dancing, or even just cleaning my room, which was always a mess. The possibilities are endless.

In the beginning, getting better took more of my time and energy than the bulimia itself. It only took minutes to throw up, but to not throw up, I had to sit there longer and convince myself not to do it. Now that I'm better, I definitely have more time than I did when I was sick. I'm physically and emotionally more free to do other things.

—Lisa, seventeen years old

It's upsetting to me that I wasted so much time and energy on anorexia.

I didn't have any real friends, I was totally isolated. I was so consumed by the whole anorexia thing that there wasn't any time or energy to give to anybody else. I also missed a huge amount of school the first half of the ninth grade because I was sick all of the time. I was so thin my body couldn't stay healthy. I always had a cold, and I was so tired I couldn't even get out of bed.

I shut myself out from the world. Food was all I could think about, and everything was focused around not eating. It's upsetting to me that I wasted so much time and energy on anorexia. I could have had many more friends, a lot more fun, and I would have gone out. I wouldn't have felt so isolated. I don't think my life would have been "wonderful and perfect" if I didn't have anorexia, but I could have done well in school and had some fun. These days, if I start slipping into the restrictive mode, I remind myself that I will miss out on so much.

—Tania, seventeen years old

It certainly is difficult to enjoy life when we are worried about how much we ate today, when our next binge will be, or where we can throw up. Eating disorders affect our relationships, our ability to concentrate, and our moods. As girls, we spend our lives being bombarded with messages about the importance of being thin—diversity of body shapes is sadly lacking on television, in the movies, and on the fashion runways. Combine this with the subtle (and sometimes not so subtle) pressures we may get from parents or peers to take off a couple of pounds, and we have a formula for an army of girls feeling dissatisfied with their bodies and dieting and eating in a way that is harmful to them. Eating disorders are also effective methods for covering up very real emotional pain and scars. A high number of us suffering from an eating disorder have had past experiences of emotional, physical, or sexual abuse. We need to work on whatever underlying issues we may have and work hard toward developing a healthy eating pattern that supports us rather than harms us.

It's time for all of us to start investing in our health and celebrating our own body types—and encouraging our friends to do the same. Getting beyond an eating disorder means seeking counseling and finding other outlets for our emotions and stress. Eating disorders are very real and should not be taken lightly. With the proper support, we can find the strength to recover and share our insights and experience with others.

I can look at it and use it—I have this experience inside of me, and maybe I can help other people.

I still have to be careful about not slipping back into anorexia. I used to have no idea of what was going on, I was in total denial. Now when I do certain things, like when I restrict what I am eating, I can immediately say, "I'm doing this to myself, this is wrong, I shouldn't do this." But it doesn't always help, sometimes I still want to restrict. It's definitely related to stress—if the stress level is high or if anything is going wrong in my life, I think, "There is something wrong with me, I need to gain control." Also, if I'm feeling bad about myself in any context, I immediately think, "I feel fat," or "I feel ugly." In the past, the immediate thing to do would be to diet so I could lose weight and look beautiful. In my mind there was this single solution to all problems: lose weight to be beautiful. I understand myself much better now, and I see my own patterns. I would like to go on and help others see this for themselves.

I believe at the very core of my being that my eating disorder will always be with me. At times I feel smothered as if there's nothing I can do to be over it completely. I feel like, "Why did this have to happen to me?" I want to get rid of it. Tell someone, "Take it away!" But, at the same time, I can look at it and use it—I have this experience inside of me, and maybe I can help other people. If I can talk to others who are suffering, that's a gift.

—Luisa, seventeen years old

Because I had such a wonderful friend and I felt so comfortable and secure, I didn't need to worry about losing weight.

From eighth to tenth grade, I went through anorexia. It was all about trying to look like everyone else around me. They were all these little nymphets, and I had matured so quickly. They were really skinny, little people, and I wanted to prove that I could look like that too because I never had. So I started counting calories and working out all the time. I ate no fat, and I had no fat on my body; it was all muscle. Of course I still felt like I was fat. I wanted to keep losing weight, and it was a triumph whenever I could. My father was supportive and proud if I lost weight, so that was a reinforcement.

My sophomore year, I met Suzanne. She and I were immediate best friends. I had never been that close to anyone in my whole life. Suzanne was slightly over-

Getting Help for Eating Problems

You are not alone! If you are struggling with an eating disorder, here are some organizations that can provide you with the support you need and deserve:

Anorexia Nervosa and Related Eating Disorders, Inc.

ANRED is a nonprofit organization that was founded in 1979 to combat eating disorders. Its website provides information about eating disorders, including definitions, statistics, warning signs, complications, and resources.

PO Box 5102. Eugene, OR 97401

phone: (503) 344-1144

website: www.anred.com

Colours of Ana

This website is about eating disorders and women of color. Published in the United Kingdom by a black woman who has suffered from eating disorders, it features research, resources, artwork, personal stories, and a forum where eating disorder sufferers can share and receive support.

website: www.coloursofana.com

The Harvard Eating Disorders Center

The Harvard Eating Disorders Center is affiliated with the Harvard Medical School and is a leading academic research center for eating disorders. The HEDC was established to expand and share knowledge about eating disorders, their detection, treatment, and prevention. The website includes definitions, facts, research, and a thorough list of web-links and organizations.

website: www.hedc.org

weight, and no matter what I did, I was always thinner than she was. She was so relaxed about food and her body that it made me forget about my food obsession. Because I had such a wonderful friend and I felt so comfortable and secure, I didn't need to worry about losing weight. It was a slow process, but it was right after meeting Suzanne that all my issues about my body started to go away. Suzanne would tell me how ridiculous I was being and say things like, "What are you doing? Eat!" It made me start questioning, "What am I doing?" Now I don't worry about what I eat,

National Eating Disorders Association

NEDA offers videos, a newsletter, conferences, workshops, a help line, and a national speakers bureau.
603 Stewart, Suite 803
Seattle, WA 98101
phone: (800) 931-2237
website: www.nationaleatingdisorders.org

Overeaters Anonymous Headquarters

This free twelve-step peer support program helps people confront and deal with compulsive overeating. Check your phone book for local chapters.
PO Box 44020, Rio Rancho, NM 87174
phone: (505) 891-2664
email: info@overeatersanonymous.org
website: www.overeatersanonymous.org

Something Fishy

This very thorough website created by a woman recovering from anorexia provides information about symptoms of eating disorders and places to get help if you have an eating problem. It also features a chat room and a very touching memorial to individuals who have died as a result of eating disorders.
website: www.something-fishy.org

and I eat pretty much whatever I want. If I see I'm getting flabby, I work out, but that's a matter of staying healthy not a matter of having to be thin. I think more about how I feel, not what I eat.

—Marissa, eighteen years old

4

Take a Good Look Down There
Menstruation, Anatomy, Orgasms, and Masturbation

We can be so goofy when it comes to discussing anything having to do with our vaginas. Clitorises, orgasms, periods, and masturbation are often whispered about like secrets or dirty words. We even use slang instead of the actual terms: "On the rag," "the curse," "raining down south," and "a red week" are all phrases used to describe menstruation, while "honeypot," "muff," "box," and "pussy" are used instead of "vagina" or "vulva." So, let's stop beating around the bush and start talking.

I always thought the vagina was just a little spot on the outside.

I realized what a vagina was for the first time when I was nine and witnessed my sister putting a tampon in. I was awestruck by watching this white cotton thing disappear between my sister's legs. I exclaimed, "Where did that go?" I had always been told, "Girls have vaginas and boys have penises," but I always thought the vagina was just a little spot on the outside. My sis enlightened me by explaining it was actually more like a cave and went inside me.

—Dorine, sixteen years old

Getting Your Period: How Big a Deal Is It?

so i excuse myself and leave the room
saying my period came early but it's not a minute too soon
i go and find the only other woman on the floor
it's the secretary sitting at the desk by the door
i ask her if she's got a tampon i can use
she says oh honey what a hassle for you sure i do you know i do
i say it ain't no hassle no it ain't no mess
right now it's the only power that i possess

—Ani DiFranco "Blood in the Boardroom," *Puddle Dive*

Most of us get our first period between the ages of nine and sixteen, the average age being twelve to fourteen. Dealing with our first menstrual cycle can mean getting involved with our vaginas on an intimate level—for some of us this is the first time we touch and examine our genitals, while others of us have already done considerable exploring. You'll also get to know your flow—when it tends to be heavy, light, or somewhere in between.

In the beginning, we may feel some awkwardness in dealing with our periods. For example, some of us have a hard time figuring out how to put in a tampon. Talking to someone we trust or carefully reading the detailed instructions in the tampon box can get us on the road to easy insertion. Some of us never use tampons and stick to pads, and some of us combine methods or find alternative ones (see the section beginning on page 100). Eventually we all find our favorite routines.

Take a trip to the "Museum of Menstruation," an online museum devoted to menstruation and women's health. It's the place to find the latest information on menstrual caps, an in-depth history of sanitary products, humorous anecdotes, art, and much, much more. www.mum.org.

I actually enjoy getting my period every month—I feel older.

I was expecting my period. I was in tenth grade, and by then most of my friends had already gotten theirs and had stopped thinking about it. I knew that it would come someday. On my fifteenth birthday, it arrived. I woke up, and I sang, "Well, happy birthday to myself," and I thought, "It's about time." I was happy. I told my mom about it, and she patted me on the back and said, "Don't forget to use your sanitary napkins." I actually enjoy getting my period every month—I feel older.

—Eisa, eighteen years old

When I got my period, my grandmother announced it in front of my huge family at dinner.

I was embarrassed; I ran into the bathroom crying. She made it seem like such a big deal, like my life was changed forever. There were things I didn't know about having my period. One day, I had to ask a friend what I should do if my pad crinkles and makes noise when I walk. She said I should cough. I realized I had lost a lot of freedom and that I felt more responsible.

—Zana, sixteen years old

Every summer, I used to try to put tampons in, but I couldn't figure it out.

It was a pain because napkins are like diapers, and I missed going swimming. I didn't know how a tampon would fit in my vagina. A friend told me to try putting some K-Y Jelly on the applicator, which really helped.

—Libby, eighteen years old

Our Bodies, the Media . . . and Fields of Daisies?

The media are no help in educating us about our sexual anatomy. The words and phrases they use to describe our bodily functions are often vague or incomprehensible. Television and print ads usually avoid terms associated with our natural functions, relying instead on phrases like, "those difficult days," "times like these," or just "those days," leaving us to figure out that they are referring to menstruation.

Ads for douching products often show young women running through fields of daisies. It looks like they're selling a vacation, not a vaginal cleanser! Douching is not about taking a vacation, it is when plain water or a diluted cleanser such as vinegar or baking soda, is inserted into the vagina to get rid of odors. And while we're on the subject, douching isn't really even necessary for healthy women—in fact, douching can wash out the vagina's natural, friendly bacteria, which are necessary for fighting infections.

When my mom got home, she celebrated with me.

I cried the first time I got my period. I was eleven, and none of my friends had gotten it yet. I felt embarrassed because that was something the older girls had. I didn't want to tell my friends. I waited to tell them until they started getting theirs. It was a little scary; I wasn't a little kid anymore, and it was a surprise. When my mom got home, she celebrated with me. She said, "It's supposed to happen. It's natural, and now you are becoming a woman." She comforted me.

—Marcela, sixteen years old

Historical Fear of Menstruation

It is an undoubted fact that meat spoils when touched by menstruating women.

—British Medical Journal, 1878

Social discomfort and confusion about menstruation are nothing new. People once feared that menstrual blood contained "potent and dangerous energy." Menstruation has been seen as everything from a punishment for sexual activity, to a sign that a woman should have formed a child and didn't, to evidence that women were simply unclean. In some cultures, menstruating women have been excluded from society—especially from any contact with religious figures. Like so many attitudes toward women's sexuality, fears about menstruation were based on ignorance, not facts.

Myth: We lose our virginity by using a tampon.

Reality: We lose our virginity through sexual intercourse.

Myth: We can't swim or exercise during our periods.

Reality: We can participate in the same activities we enjoy during the rest of the month. While some of us barely notice symptoms during our periods, others have cramps and/or premenstrual symptoms that might make us not want to exercise. Exercise won't hurt, and it may even help us feel better.

Myth: We lose tons of blood with every period.

Reality: A typical menstrual period involves blood loss of four to six tablespoons (two to three ounces). That's it!

Every girl must have an embarrassing period story.
Like the time I wore a white skirt and got my "friend" or the time I forgot to bring supplies and had to ask to borrow from my lab partner. As horrifying as it feels at the time, you realize soon enough that it's part of girldom, and actually girls jump to help another in need. So there is nothing to fear when asking to borrow a tampon, and no one actually notices that your jacket has been wrapped around your waist all day.

—Cassie, eighteen years old

Notes on Menstrual Cycles

A menstrual cycle is the time from the first day of one period to the first day of our next period. A "regular" menstrual cycle varies between twenty and thirty-six days. Typically, the menstrual flow lasts three to eight days (the average is five days). When we first begin menstruating, it may take a while for our menstrual cycles to become regular, but after a while, a regular cycle should kick in—usually after six to eighteen months.

The monthly cycle we go through is the result of sex hormones that are continuously produced during the reproductive part of our lives—meaning the time of our lives when we can have a baby. This life phase starts with our first period and goes until we begin menopause, usually around age fifty-one, when our bodies enter the non-reproductive stage of life. Though the flow of menstrual "blood" (actually a mixture of blood, mucus, and parts of the lining of the uterus) is the most obvious part of the cycle for us, our bodies are actually cycling through changes during the entire month. There are three main players in our menstrual cycle: the hypothalamus, the pituitary gland, and the ovaries. These three perform a sort of dance within our bodies each month by signaling to each other with hormones, which are carried from one part of the body to the other through the blood.

The monthly dance goes like this: The ovaries produce fluctuating amounts of estrogen and progesterone throughout the month. These hormones affect the hypothalamus, which sends signals to the pituitary gland, which in turn produces the follicle stimulating hormone (FSH) and luteinizing hormone (LH). It is the FSH and LH that signal follicles in the ovaries to ripen and eventually release an egg. The egg travels down to the uterus, which has been slowly building up a lining as a direct result of the increasing progesterone levels from the follicles. When the egg is not fertilized by sperm, LH tells the follicles that released the egg to slow down the production of progesterone, which in turn triggers the shedding of the uterus lining—resulting in the period flow (and a run to the drugstore for supplies).

The following chart illustrates the monthly hormonal tango that takes place in the female body:

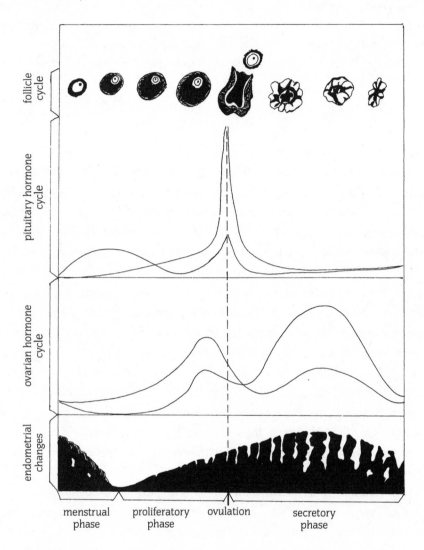

follicle cycle

pituitary hormone cycle

ovarian hormone cycle

endometrial changes

| menstrual phase | proliferatory phase | ovulation | secretory phase |

Understanding our menstrual cycles may seem complicated, but knowing some of the basics is an important step in getting to know our bodies and keeping them healthy. One very helpful thing we can do is keep a journal for a few months, noting the changes our bodies go through each day. We'll notice that besides getting our periods we have various secretions from our vaginas (with changes in color, texture, taste, and amount of wetness). We may have changes in our breasts (their sensitivity and size), as well as fluctuations in our general physical and emotional states. All of these fluctuations make sense when we realize how many hormones cycle through our bodies each month!

When Our Periods Are Irregular

Irregular menstrual periods are periods that occur too frequently (twice a month or more) or too infrequently (less often than every three months, or not at all). Our menstrual flow may also be unusually heavy or light. Many things can cause us to have irregular periods—for example, we may not be getting the correct amount of nutrition, or our bodies may be producing too much of a certain hormone. Irregular periods may be a sign that something serious is going on, or may not. We should consult a doctor if we frequently have irregular cycles. Reasons for irregular periods or for skipping a period include:

- Pregnancy
- Too little body fat
- Dieting
- Anorexia nervosa
- Stress or emotional factors
- Heavy athletic training
- Previous use of birth control pills
- Use of some drugs
- Hormonal imbalance
- Cysts or tumors
- Premature menopause

I started my period so much later than all my friends, and it never became regular.

Last year, I was diagnosed with a hormone imbalance called polycystic ovary condition. At first it was really hard for me to hear this because it made me feel like something was wrong with me. Periods are such a big deal in your early teens, and I didn't feel like a part of that. Also, I have acne, which can be a symptom of this hormone imbalance, and that really sucks. I don't feel bad about it now, though, because it just doesn't seem like a big deal. I don't even think about it much. I take the pill to regulate my menstrual cycle, and who cares about my hormones?

—Amy, eighteen years old

Pads and Tampons . . . and Some Alternatives

During our menstruating life, we will most likely spend more than $2,000 on sanitary pads and/or tampons. It's a big business—where did it all begin?

Before the advent of the disposable sanitary products we take for granted in their brightly colored boxes on drugstore shelves, women mostly used material like soft wool and flannel to soak up their menstrual flow. The material would then be washed, wrung out, and hung to dry before being reused.

During the first world war, army nurses began using bandaging materials from first-aid kits to absorb blood during their periods. They found it worked better than the cotton rags and towels most women had been using before. After the war, the

Toxic Shock Syndrome

Toxic shock syndrome (TSS) made news headlines in the 1980s when otherwise healthy menstruating women suddenly died from the disease. TSS is believed to be caused by a toxin produced by the bacteria that thrive in a dry vaginal environment. Using tampons that are highly absorbent can increase the risk of this bacteria multiplying in the vagina. Symptoms are sudden high fever, vomiting, diarrhea, fainting, dizziness, and/or a sunburn-like rash. Today, every box of tampons contains information on the dangers of TSS and how to avoid it.

Knowing about TSS does not mean we need to stop using tampons. Remember, TSS is an extremely rare disease. Our chances of developing this illness are very small, especially if we take the following precautions:

- Change tampons every four to six hours.
- Use the least absorbent tampon possible to meet the needs of our menstrual flow.
- Switch between pads and tampons during our period.

Kimberly-Clark company decided to sell the material as sanitary pads, calling them Kotex. At the time, Kimberly-Clark had difficulty marketing Kotex because people did not talk openly about menstruation.[1]

In 1936, tampons were introduced to the public as "a comfort never known before." Tampons were promoted as having "no belts, no pins, no pads, no odor." Today tampons make up a $718 million industry.[2] However, tampons can cause vaginal irritation if the menstrual flow is very light and the vagina is dry. When this happens, we should use lower-absorbency tampons or switch to pads.

Some women are concerned about the chlorine bleaches used in the processing of pads and tampons. Chlorine makes paper products white, and we associate whiteness with cleanliness. But the chlorine chemicals can be dangerous to the environment (and if you think about it, we really don't want chemicals near or inside our vaginas). Some health food stores carry "natural cotton" brands; however, they may not be unbleached, so be sure to check the labels. Look for them in your drugstore or health food store, and if they don't carry them, feel free to suggest that they do.

One alternative is nondisposable unbleached cotton menstrual pads and panty liners. Those of use who are interested in eco-friendly alternatives can check out Eco Logique Inc. It sells nondisposable unbleached cotton menstrual pads and panty liners as well as sponges and menstrual cups. For more information, visit www.ecologique.com or call (800) 680-9739.

Though not well known, there are some innovative alternatives to tampons and pads: Natural sponges, or sea sponges (not to be confused with the synthetic ones you use to wash your dishes!), work like tampons. Used in a size fitted to the vagina, the sponge is dampened and inserted into the vagina with a finger. The damp sponge takes the shape of your vagina and eliminates the dryness problem sometimes caused by tampons. When the sponge is full, you pull it out, wash and wring it out, and reinsert. Sponges can save you money but can also be tricky (there have been cases where the sponge has gotten stuck and required removal by a doctor). Some women tie a string to the sponge for easier extraction, but this is not recommended because the string is a magnet for external bacteria. It is important to boil sponges in water before using for the first time and to store them in a clean, dry place between periods. Keep in mind that sea sponges are not approved by the Federal Drug Administration and therefore are not labeled as menstrual-flow absorbers.

In 1998, 7 billion tampons and 13 billion sanitary pads and their packaging were disposed of in the United States—that's a lot of waste![3] An environmentally friendly alternative, menstrual cups (also known as menstrual caps), are worn in the vagina and catch menstrual blood before it leaks out of the body. The Keeper is a reusable menstrual cup, and, like the sponge, is removed regularly to wash out the menstrual blood and is then reinserted. The Instead brand, introduced in 1996, is a disposable menstrual cup. The Diva Cup is another option. All of these devices hold more of your menstrual flow than a sponge or tampon. By trial and error, you begin to learn when it is full and needs to be removed, washed, and reinserted.

For more information on The Keeper, go to www.softcup.com, and for Diva Cup information, check out www.divacup.com. You may be able to find Instead products at your local drugstore, or call (800) INSTEAD.

Premenstrual Syndrome: Real or Imagined?

Before our periods, we may feel bloated, super-hungry, crampy, achey, nauseated, or just plain upset—symptoms called premenstrual syndrome (PMS). Not all of us experience PMS; some of us barely notice a difference between when we are having our period and when we are not, and glide through our menstruating days comfortably. PMS symptoms may have to do with hormonal changes around our menstrual cycles. Symptoms, such as cramps, usually last for only a day or two. But some of us may experience discomfort starting up to two weeks before our period and lasting throughout our period. Those of us who have severe symptoms that interfere with daily life may not have PMS but PMDD (premenstrual dysphoric disorder) instead. PMDD is treatable, so if you experience depression, anxiety, or extreme irritability before or during your period, you should seek medical advice.

Upwards of 75 percent of women report some physical or emotional symptoms before their periods.[1] A huge number and range of symptoms have been said to be related to our periods: more than 150 different symptoms in all! They range from your run-of-the-mill muscle pain to extreme symptoms, like epilepsy or suicidal thoughts. Such severe symptoms have never been medically linked to menstruation. Yet, in a court of law, PMS has been used as an explanation for murder. Some of us think PMS is all in our heads because there is little reliable research that gives us a definite answer about what it is.

Those of us who experience PMS don't sit around and debate whether or not it's real and what the precise symptoms are. Instead, we seek remedies for the symptoms and try not to let them interfere with our lives. It has been shown that stress is a trigger for PMS—so managing stress while cutting down on caffeine, eating a healthy diet (with lots of whole grains, fruits, and vegetables), drinking lots of water, and taking multivitamins may decrease PMS.

My period doesn't affect me much at all.

When I'm in a bad mood, sometimes my mom will think it's PMS, and I'll know it has nothing to do with it. I'll say, "Don't blame that." I don't believe my period bothers me that much.

—Gina, seventeen years old

PMS totally exists.

People who say it doesn't are full of baloney. Every person I know gets so nasty around their period. My best friend will start flipping out at the drop of a hat. If someone accidentally brushes her foot to pick up their pen, she'll freak out: "Why are you touching me? Don't touch me, I hate you!" And she'll storm out. She storms out of classrooms more than anybody else I know. When I'm feeling irritable, I never make the connection with my period, and neither does she. But when we get our period, it's like, "Oh, no wonder. Aah. No wonder you were being so nasty."

—Leah, seventeen years old

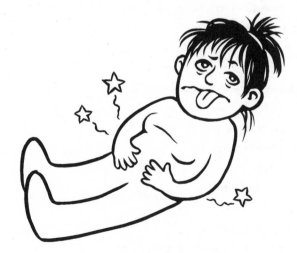

The Curse

Sometimes, I call it a curse:
No pad in my purse,
one week early, caught in class.
The dash to the bathroom only finds
empty or broken dispenser machines . . .
The cold walk home, coat tied around
my waist, shame blooming
in a stubborn stain.
Or the pain—
like a planet's inside me, pulling
against me, out of phase.
Sometimes, I call it being "on the rag":
The first two days, the drag
of sleep is like waves upon me—
I am little more than body, curled to a heap,
and the bed's so deep and black and sure.
Or those days when, just before I bleed,
each month I'm drawn
to department stores, to "Women's Wear,"
to bathing suits, then dressing rooms
with mirrors all around and greenish,
mean fluorescent lighting.
I always believe the fun-house mirror
in my brain, that tells me:
"You are ugly, greasy, stinking, fat!"
And I end up buying
only that. Yeah, sometimes I wish I could
simply be a man.

But I am a woman
tuned to my body, always turning—
fertile and ever better learning
to map myself,
as tides.

Besides,

men have their cycles, too,

cursed by not knowing that they do.

–Gillian White

Getting to Know Your Anatomy

Those pictures in health ed of the female anatomy were always confusing to me.

I had a hard time figuring out where those things were on me. It didn't seem real. And when I looked at myself, I didn't look like those hand-drawn pictures. But I felt embarrassed to ask because I felt like I should just know. Last year, my mom gave me a copy of Our Bodies, Ourselves *and it completely educated me. Me and my girlfriends can spend hours in front of it, poring over the information.*

—Talia, 17 years old

It's obviously a whole lot easier for boys to be familiar with their penises than for us to know our vaginas, vulvas, and clitorises. We need a mirror just to get a good look down there. Sometimes we are pretty clueless when it comes to this part of our bodies. (Do you know your major labia from your minor labia?) Get to know your body: Take a look at this picture of the vagina and surrounding area; now, if you're in the mood, check out your own in a handy-dandy mirror.

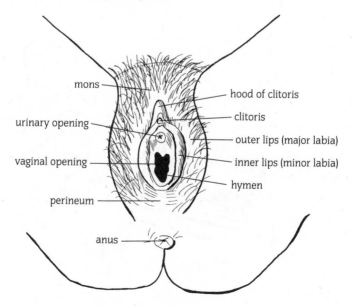

Pelvic Exams: The Journey to the Gynecologist

I'm afraid to go to the gynecologist.
I don't want someone staring at me naked, putting things in my vagina, and shining lights on me. It makes me really nervous, even though I should go.
—Talisha, eighteen years old

Many of us are nervous about going to the gynecologist, especially the first time. Lack of straightforward information about the exam can lead to fear or embarrassment, which may stop some of us from going to this important checkup. But pelvic exams are an important way to ensure that we are healthy. They are also a great opportunity to ask an expert questions we may have about our health and sexuality. It is recommended that all girls have a pelvic exam by age eighteen or when they start having sex (anal, oral, or vaginal). If we are sexually active, having a yearly pelvic exam by a gynecologist will help to tell us if we have a sexually transmitted infection (STI). Some STIs cannot be detected by the exam but require a specific test. If we think we have engaged in activity that puts us at risk for an STI, we should request to be tested.

A pelvic exam should be relatively painless. By getting one, we can feel proud that we did something important for our health. Nurse practitioners, physician's assistants, and doctors perform pelvic exams. When making an appointment, we can ask for a

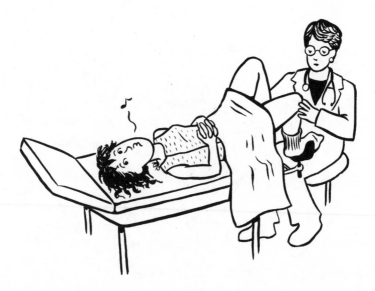

The Hymen

The hymen is a thin tissue that stretches across part of the opening of the vagina. Usually, at the time of first intercourse, the hymen stretches and/or tears, and there may be a small amount of blood. An intact hymen was historically used as proof that a woman was a virgin. Some groups believe that a woman's virginity is evidence of her purity and that she should remain a virgin until marriage. In some societies, if a groom-to-be found out that his bride did not have an intact hymen, she could be returned to her family, humiliated, physically abused, or even put to death![1] However, the condition of the hymen is an inaccurate indicator for past sexual behavior. Some women are born without a hymen, or it may be broken through physical activities or the insertion of a finger or object in the vagina. Imagine all the women who suffered from the mistaken belief that a virgin had to have an intact hymen.

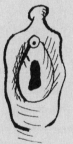 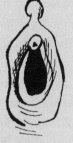 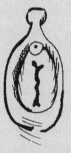

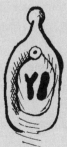 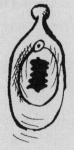 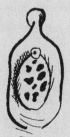

some hymen variations

woman to examine us. The examiner should help us feel relaxed and explain what she is doing. We can ask any questions (she has certainly heard them all before). And if we do not feel as if the examiner is respecting what we say or how we feel, we can leave. We can also bring a friend, our mom, or a sister if that makes us more comfortable.

The Exam: What to Expect

- You lie down on an examination table wearing a paper gown or cloth robe. You place your feet into open stirrups at the end of the table. The stirrups are far apart so that your legs are spread open when your feet are in place. The examiner has you scoot your butt to the edge of the table. This is the examining position. It's awkward and you may feel vulnerable, but it's a convenient position for the health care provider to do the exam.
- The provider shines a light at your vulva and vagina and begins the examination.
- A metal or plastic speculum is put into your vagina and gently opened so that the doctor or nurse can check inside. It may feel a little uncomfortable when the speculum is opened, but it should not hurt. If it does, make sure you say so.
- Pap smear: Usually a thin wooden spatula or a tiny cyto brush is put into your vagina to take some cells from your cervix. Pap smears are sent to a lab to make sure there is no abnormal cell growth. This should not hurt either.
- The examiner will put two gloved fingers inside your vagina and push down on your abdomen to check your organs, such as your uterus and ovaries. When the doctor or nurse finds your ovaries, it may hurt for a few seconds.
- Many practitioners will also put a gloved finger into your anus to check the area between the vagina and the rectum. Yes, this feels awkward (and sometimes like you want to have a bowel movement) but it lasts just a few seconds.
- Breast exam: Your breasts are examined—by eye and touch—for lumps or discharge from the nipples. This may be done before or after the pelvic exam.

That's it! The more relaxed you can be during an exam, the easier it will be—for you and for the examiner. If you are feeling tense, take some deep breaths or hum a tune.

It was great to have the gynecologist say that I was really healthy down there. All girls should go.

I was really nervous about the exam because she put this big plastic thing in my vagina. But she explained everything to me, movement by movement. "You see

Your Vagina Is Your Friend

Here are some enlightening books that can help us get more familiar with our bodies, our health, and the changes we are going through:

The Black Women's Health Book: Speaking for Ourselves edited by Evelyn C. White, Seattle: Seal Press, 1994.

Body and Soul: The Black Women's Guide to Physical Health and Emotional Well-Being edited by Linda Villarosa, New York: HarperPerennial, 1994.

It's a Girl Thing: How to Stay Healthy, Safe, and In Charge by Mavis Jukes, New York: Alfred A. Knopf, 1996.

It's Perfectly Normal: A Book About Changing Bodies, Growing Up, Sex, and Sexual Health by Robie H. Harris, Cambridge, MA: Candlewick Press, 2004.

The Lesbian Health Book: Caring for Ourselves edited by Jocelyn White, MD, and Marissa C. Martínez, Seattle: Seal Press, 1997.

Our Bodies, Ourselves for the New Century: A Book By and For Women by the Boston Women's Health Book Collective, New York: Simon & Schuster, 1998.

Period: A Girl's Guide to Menstruation by JoAnn Gardner-Loulan and Bonnie Worthen, Minnetonka, MN: Book Peddlers, 2001.

The Period Book: Everything You Don't Want to Ask (But Need to Know) by Karen Gravelle, et al., New York: Walker & Company, 1996.

Salud!: A Latina's Guide to Total Health by Jane L. Delgado, New York: Rayo, 2002.

Sex for One: The Joy of Selfloving by Betty Dodson, New York: Crown Trade Paperbacks, 1996.

Women's Bodies, Women's Wisdom: Creating Physical and Emotional Health and Healing by Christiane Northup, New York: Bantam Books, 1998.

this, I'm going to put it in your vagina, and it might be cold . . ." "This might feel funny, but just relax." I always thought that gynecologists were for older people. I think that parents should talk to their kids. My mom wouldn't take me to a gynecologist because she was sure I was a virgin. But I'm glad I decided to go on my own. It was great to have the gynecologist say that I was really healthy down there. All girls should go.

—Samia, **eighteen years old**

Orgasms: Our Bodies Rejoice

I always thought you had to be screaming to have an orgasm.

All the stories I heard were of women yelling. I recently realized I've been having orgasms through masturbation. I talked to my cousin about it, and she explained that an orgasm can feel like a release of tension and a warm trembling feeling, which is what I have been experiencing.

—Magdah, **sixteen years old**

There is a lot of mystery around the female orgasm. We usually don't get to talk openly about this topic on our own. So let's get to it! During an orgasm, sexual tension that has built up in our bodies is released in a series of rhythmic muscular contractions in the vagina, uterus, and rectum. The contractions are very fast, less than one-tenth of a second apart. Orgasms can be mild or strong, a mild one having just three to four contractions, a longer and stronger one having twelve or more contractions. Some of us describe a feeling of very comfortable warmth and sudden relaxation of our entire body during an orgasm. Our experiences may range from explosive to mellow waves. And unlike guys, we can have many orgasms in a row.

I was surprised—I had no idea that such a thing could happen to you.

Considering all the sex I had, it's amazing that I never had an orgasm until I met Ricky. With Ricky it was different because we both wanted to have sex, and I was comfortable with him. The first time I had an orgasm during sex, my legs started shaking. I felt like I was seeing stars—there were these flashes of little lights, and my whole body was tingling. It was kind of scaring me because it felt too wonderful. After that, we practiced giving each other orgasms and it was great. I would get satisfaction out of it as well as him. I was surprised—I had no idea that such a thing could happen to you. I felt refreshed and I would go to sleep relieved. Orgasms are better than a massage or a workout.

—Marilyn, **eighteen years old**

I haven't had orgasms every time I've had sex, but it feels good every time.
It's better, though, when you do have an orgasm. The guys I would want to get to know better are the guys who know how to satisfy me before they satisfy themselves. It doesn't take much for them to come, and it's more fun if you can play with each other instead of "Okay, it's over" and falling asleep. If he doesn't talk to me after we've had sex and turns his back to me saying, "Oh, I'm tired," that's the worst thing.
—Shirleen, seventeen years old

Clitoris: Its Only Function Is Female Pleasure

Myth: The clitoris is a female mini-penis.

Reality: The clitoris is not the female version of the penis. Maybe because there is no male equivalent or because in embryos, the same tissue that becomes a clitoris for girls becomes a penis for boys, people make the mistake of referring to the clitoris in this way.

The clitoris has no reproductive or urinary functions; it's purely for pleasure. Though small, it is one of the most sensitive areas of our genitals and gets slightly enlarged when stimulated. It is located outside the vagina, just beneath the point where the top of the inner lips meet. The size and appearance of the clitoris vary from female to female. The only directly visible part of the clitoris is the head (the clitoral glans), which looks like a tiny knob.

So I made a vow to get to know what was going on down there.
I was doing a ridiculous quiz in Cosmopolitan, *and I realized that I had no clue about my clitoris. I didn't know what it looked like, where exactly it was, or what it was supposed to do. So I made a vow to get to know what was going on "down there." I looked at myself in a mirror and started touching myself. I definitely noticed some parts were more sensitive than others. Then I looked in my sister's biology book and saw a picture of female anatomy. I didn't masturbate to orgasm for a few months, but just exploring felt good.*

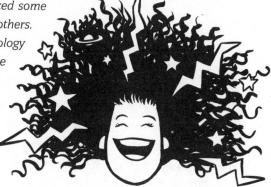

—Zana, seventeen years old

G-Spot: The Hot Spot?

A female pleasure point, the G-spot (Grafenberg spot) has made headlines in recent years. Fantastic stories appeared about a mysterious spot in the vagina that, when located and pressed, would bring a woman to orgasm, even resulting in female ejaculation. While some women searched for or experimented with their G-spots, others debated whether this spot actually existed.

In reality, this spot was old news. In the 1950s, Dr. Ernest Grafenberg (Mr. G-spot) wrote about what many women knew since the beginning of time—that stimulating the front wall of the vagina could trigger the expulsion of a thin fluid from the urethra. This bodily fluid, which is not urine, can amount to anywhere from a few drops to more than a cup! While there remain some skeptics, there is evidence that anywhere from 10–40 percent of females have this release during orgasm.[2] If we insert a finger into our vagina, we can locate the G-spot by gently pressing upward in a twelve o'clock direction. For some of us, stimulation of the G-spot enhances sexual pleasure and can lead to orgasm.

How Do We Have Orgasms?

The two most common ways to achieve an orgasm (or climax or come) are:

1. By stimulation of the clitoris
2. By pressure on the vagina walls (for example, through intercourse or inserting a finger)

Some of us prefer a clitoral orgasm, some of us prefer vaginal—both are groovy. The time it takes to reach orgasm is different for all of us. On average, it takes longer for us to reach orgasm than it does for a guy, but this is not always true. To reach orgasm with a partner, we often need to talk to them and tell them what feels good. We may need to tell our partner to touch our clitoris, as intercourse alone does not bring all of us to orgasm. It may be harder to reach orgasm if we've been drinking or taking drugs, are low in energy, have our mind on something else, or feel worried or tense.

One time I was with this guy and we found an article in a magazine about the G-spot.
We tried to find my G-spot. It took a while, but when we did find the right spot it was really great.

—Felicia, eighteen years old

Masturbation: Pleasure of Our Own

Masturbation means touching our own genitals for pleasure. There is a ridiculous notion that girls don't masturbate, but most of us do. In a study of women ages eighteen to thirty-six, 75 percent said they had masturbated to the point of orgasm during their teenage years.[3] So don't be shy! Masturbation means we can get sexual satisfaction without having to be with a partner.

There is a wide range of masturbation experience among girls: We may have had an orgasm through masturbation before the age of ten, we may have just experimented yesterday, or we may have never tried. We have the freedom to decide if we want to masturbate or not. It's fine if we are not interested in masturbating, but if we are interested, it's never too late to try. The clitoris is extremely receptive to touch, and with experimentation we can reach orgasm. Exploring our bodies is a healthy and natural thing to do; even babies masturbate. When we understand our own bodies well, it can increase our pleasure with a partner because we know what turns us on. As a wise motto says, "Learn it yourself before taking it on the road."

Myth: You can lose your virginity by masturbating.
Reality: You lose your virginity when you have sexual intercourse for the first time.

Myth: Lots of boys masturbate. Hardly any girls do.
Reality: Boys may feel more comfortable talking about masturbation, but three out of four girls are likely to masturbate.

Masturbation can be a natural way to discover something about yourself.
For me, masturbating didn't occur naturally. I bought a medical book at age fourteen and learned by reading the description in the book. I think that masturbation can be a natural way to discover something about yourself. It's good to try it at least. For boys there are so many jokes about masturbating, while for girls it is more of a closed subject. But to talk deeply about it, I don't think boys have it any easier.

—Yvette, seventeen years old

I think masturbation is a good and healthy thing to do, unless it takes up all your time—that's not great.

When I was eleven, one of my friends taught me. She was spending the night at my house, and she showed me how she masturbated. I thought it was fascinating and began experimenting myself.

—Tara, seventeen years old

Sexual Fantasies: Having Fun with Daydreams

I love to have fantasies about a cute person I saw on the bus or a guy I just met on my block.

Of course, I could masturbate while reading my math book, but fantasies add a lot of pleasure to it.

—Norma, sixteen years old

Freud's View on Female Orgasms: An Outrage from the Guy Who Said We All Really Want Penises Anyway!

In the early 1900s, Sigmund Freud's theories about women's sexuality included the idea that a girl's orgasm was clitoral in childhood and should become vaginally oriented as she matured. He stated that the only "mature" orgasm was through vaginal intercourse. If a woman could only have a clitoral orgasm, it meant she was "frigid" and immature. Many women were baffled about their own body's ability to reach orgasm because of Freud's inaccurate teaching. In reality, most women reach orgasm through clitoral stimulation and not through vaginal pressure. These days, Freud's theories about female sexuality are rejected by the medical world, and women rejoice in the pleasures of clitoral orgasms.

The clitoral orgasm is like your whole body is this electrical storm.

—Marilyn, eighteen years old

Sexual fantasies help us have sexual pleasure. Fantasies can be a safe and controlled way to experiment with sexuality in the privacy of our own mind. Fantasies also help us to create arousal and reach orgasm. We can replay sexual situations in our mind or imagine fooling around with a person we have a crush on. Thinking of what we might do or would enjoy doing sexually can make us more comfortable with sexual situations with a partner. Sometimes we are not comfortable with what we are fantasizing about. If our fantasies disturb us, we can talk about them to a counselor or someone we trust.

Know the Facts, Have Fun, and Be Healthy

The more we know about our bodies, the more we can love them. Our period does not ever have to be considered a "curse." Once we become familiar with the harmony of our hormones, we can appreciate the mastery behind our menstrual cycles. Orgasms and masturbation do not need to be great mysteries that we can discuss only in whispers—they are a part of our sexuality to celebrate, and we have a right to know the facts. Keeping yourself healthy, both mentally and physically, means getting informed (and getting those pelvic exams!). Our natural state is feeling comfortable and at ease in our birthday suits. So take the time to get to know your body and feel proud of your female form.

Taking Back Our Health

Being informed about our bodies is being in charge. Contact these organizations to learn more about women's health issues:

Advocates for Youth
200 M Street NW, Suite 750
Washington, D.C. 20030
phone: (202) 419-3420
website: www.advocatesforyouth.org

American Social Health Association
PO Box 13827
Research Triangle Park, NC 27709
phone: (919) 361-8400
website: www.ashastd.org

Black Women's Health Imperative
600 Pennsylvania Avenue SE, Suite 310
Washington, D.C. 20003
phone: (202) 548-4000
website: www.blackwomenshealth.org

Boston Women's Health Book Collective
34 Plympton Street
Boston, MA 02118
phone: (617) 451-3666
website: www.ourbodiesourselves.org

Engender Health
440 9th Avenue
New York, NY 10001
phone: (212) 561-8000
website: www.engenderhealth.org

National Alliance for Hispanic Health

1501 16th Street NW
Washington, D.C. 20036
phone: (202) 387-5000
website: www.hispanichealth.org

National Lesbian and Gay Health Association

1407 S Street NW
Washington, D.C. 20009
phone: (202) 939-7880

National Women's Health Network

514 10th Street NW, Suite 400
Washington, D.C. 20004
phone: (202) 628-7814
website: www.nwhn.org

Native American Women's Health Education Resource Center

PO Box 572
Lake Andes, SD 57356
phone: (605) 487-7072
website: www.nativeshop.org

Planned Parenthood Federation

phone: (800) 230-PLAN (connects you to clinic nearest you)
website: www.plannedparenthood.org

Sex Information and Educational Council for K–12

130 West 42nd Street, Suite 350
New York, NY 10036
phone: (212) 819-9770
website: www.siecus.org

5

Coming to Terms
with Our Sexuality

Sex: a tiny word with a huge meaning. We are told to do the right thing when it comes to sex, but how are we defining "sex," and what is the "right" thing? Is sex just intercourse, and abstinence just not having intercourse? That is what some sex education classes teach, but certainly anal and oral sex are just as intimate and can put us at risk for sexually transmitted infections if we do not use protection. Sex (and for the purpose of this chapter, we mean vaginal, oral, or anal) is often treated awkwardly and with little real communication, yet more than half of us have sexual intercourse by our eighteenth birthday and most of the rest of us are interested in the issue.

When it comes to sex, many of us are left to struggle through the choices alone or with questionable information. We are supposed to be responsible about sex, but then we turn on the television and see lots of folks being *irresponsible* about it. And if we are lesbian or bisexual, we rarely get to see ourselves represented at all.

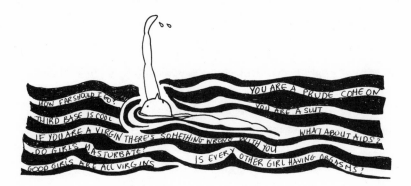

We encounter the glamorous side of sex in movies, magazines, television shows, romance novels, popular music, and love songs: On an average soap opera alone, unmarried couples refer to sex two to three times an hour,[1] and music videos flash images of sexy people gyrating to thumping beats. But have you noticed that there is almost never any mention of contraception or pregnancy? We are left to fill in the blanks after the lights and the music fade. Where's the fumbling, the condoms, the worrying, the sweaty palms, and the mishaps? Where's the real stuff? It's hard to know what to think of our own experiences when there are so few frank portrayals about the realities of sex.

Recent headlines have highlighted a new trend of casual sex among young adults: "friends with benefits" (fooling around with friends with no strings attached), "hooking up," and the unsettling new fad of suburban middle-schoolers regularly engaging in oral sex as a substitute for going all the way.[2] Yet, these headlines are based on small samples and anecdotal evidence and can neither be confirmed nor denied since no accurate data has been collected.[3] Instead, we are left with more hype and speculation, as well as a continued lack of open discussion around our sexuality. Whether or not we are sexually active, arming ourselves with the facts keeps sex in perspective as a healthy, safe, and enjoyable part of life for us to explore.

People said, When you look in the mirror after you lose your virginity, you will feel different.
That is so silly—no, I didn't look any different the next day.
—Ann, seventeen years old

I feel like I make love now even though I haven't had sex.
The actual act doesn't change that much; it's more that it can mean disease, pregnancy, and emotions being mixed up. There is so much pressure put on that one act.
—Talisa, sixteen years old

I think sex will change me because it is special and I'll be more of a woman.
It is opening yourself up to someone you love a lot. It's like having a castle with a fortress that no one has ever entered. It is an intimacy that changes you. I want to be with someone I love because otherwise I think I would suffer. A lot of people think I'm old to be a virgin. But people also think girls who have had sex are promiscuous. My father says when you fall in love, it's to marry. I don't think you have to marry the person, but love is important when it comes to sex.
—Carla, eighteen years old

I know girls who will do anything for a guy.

In my dorm, there are girls who will do anything for certain guys on the foot-ball team. I think that makes them feel important or something, being connected to a popular guy. For me, I would never do anything where I don't feel like I am being respected. It's fine to do whatever turns you on, in my opinion, but only if it is mutu-ally satisfying.

—Tyler, nineteen years old

What I really want is to know that a person is spending time with me because they like me, not just because of the sex.

For a while in high school it didn't really matter to me who I slept with. I went through this phase where it was just having the relationship—not the person—that was important. I came to realize that none of them had meant anything to me, and that I was just trying to gain self-confidence. I was looking for someone else to make me feel good. Somewhere in my head I was trying to equate "He will sleep with me" with "I must be pretty." At some point, I realized that this wasn't true and that what I really want is to know that a person is spending time with me because they like me, not just because of the sex. Now, when I see a close friend being careless about sex, I find that I want to protect them and spare them from the pain.

—Toni, eighteen years old

Having Your Bases Covered: There's More Than One Kind of Sex

The confusion about what is considered sex is illustrated by former President Bill Clinton's 1998 announcement, "I did not have sexual relations with that woman"—implying that the oral sex he later admitted to having with Monica Lewinsky was not really sex. There is even a lack of clarity among health care workers. In a 1999 email survey of seventy-two health educators, 30 percent responded that oral sex was abstinent behavior and 29 percent responded that mutual masturbation was not abstinent behavior.[4] When the experts are not sure how to define the term "sex," then where does that leave us? Without honest information, we can be led to believe that sexual contact outside of intercourse is less risky, not valid, or "no big deal," but this is not the case.

Oral sex is genital-to-mouth contact (cunnilingus or "going down" on a woman, fellatio or "giving head" or a "blow job" to a man), which may or may not lead to an orgasm for the female or male who is receiving it. While oral sex is more common, some women also try out and engage in anal intercourse. Anal sex (sodomy), usually ignored in sex ed classes and often considered taboo, is when the penis is inserted into the partner's anus. It may lead to an orgasm for the male who is doing the penetrating; anal sex alone rarely leads to an orgasm for the partner who is receiving it. If done with too much force, anal sex can be painful and tear the delicate tissues of the rectum. Both anal and oral sex may be part of sexual foreplay that leads to vaginal intercourse, or they can be the main show.

Outercourse is sex play without vaginal intercourse. A more narrow definition of outercourse is sex play with no penetration at all—oral, anal, or vaginal. Outercourse can completely satisfy both partners and take pressure off both parties by taking intercourse (and the risk involved) out of the equation.

As with all forms of sex, we should participate only if we are enjoying it too! And we need to honor any emotions we may feel when engaging in an intimate activity like oral or anal sex, touching each others' genitals or breasts, removing clothing, etc. All of these acts are a decision that may need some forethought. We also need to keep in mind that if a partner has an STI, we are putting ourselves at risk with any contact with their bodily fluids. And the risk of transmission is higher with anal sex than with other sexual activities because the delicate tissue around the rectum can tear easily. See the next chapter, "Being in Charge of Our Sexuality," to read about condoms, dental dams, and other ways to keep sex safe.

Here is the bottom line: Do not let anyone convince you that sexual contact such as oral or anal sex is not "real" sex or is automatically safe. What we do is a choice, and the more we make it our own choice, the more satisfying it will be.

I think you can be a virgin technically but not be what I would consider "pure."

In today's society, there is a great misunderstanding of what abstinence is. It's crazy that some of my friends believe as long as they don't have actual intercourse that they are "pure" and not at risk for catching an STI. Unfortunately, some of them have learned the hard way that if they have anal or oral sex, they have to deal with STIs.

—Lucia, nineteen years old

Many teen women get little or no pleasure from sexual intercourse because their partners do not know how to give them pleasure. Outercourse helps partners learn about their bodies and how to give themselves and each other sexual pleasure.

—Planned Parenthood

My boyfriend keeps asking me about having oral sex. I like fooling around, but a blow job seems like a big step, and I'm not sure I'm ready yet.

—Chrissy, sixteen years old

Deciding to Be Sexual: You Say When

What we think about sex is tied to many things, including what our friends are doing, romantic ideas about love, our family's viewpoint, what we see in the movies and on television, and the mixed messages we receive from society. Trying to formulate our own feelings about what sex and sexuality mean to us is not easy. Deciding whether or not to have sex is even more difficult. The following list gives an idea of some of the common reasons we choose to have sex:

- Expectations: For some of us, there is an expectation that sex will change us or our relationship. For example: "If I have sex, I will be a real woman and more mature," "I'll be more popular after I have sex," or "Sex will bring us closer together." Having sex will not cause us to fall in love or change our maturity level.
- Pressure: We often feel pressure to have sex. Extreme pressure, when physical force is involved, is rape, and clearly does not leave us with a choice. However, pressure also comes from our own desire to please others, which as girls we have been encouraged to do. For example, our partner tells us that it's time or that all our friends are doing it. Trying to please others can lead to disappointment because we are not choosing sex for ourselves.
- Love: We may love our partner and decide with them to have sex. This can be a positive experience. Sex can be another way of expressing our love. However, we don't need sex to prove that we are in love. Sometimes sex and love get mixed up with each other. For example, "If you really loved me, you'd sleep with me," or "I feel guilty for sleeping with him because I wasn't in love." We may really be in love, but that may or may not mean we are ready to have sex.
- Curiosity: Some of us wonder what sex is like and want to try it out for ourselves. Wondering about sex may not be reason enough to decide it's the right time; we need to factor in the circumstances and whether we are ready to deal with sex emotionally and physically. Curiosity can lead to a positive sexual experience if the right partner, open communication, thoughtfulness, and safer sex measures are involved.

- Feelings/Desires: Sex can fulfill a desire that is aroused in us by our thoughts or physical stimulation. In the heat of the moment, sex can be a temptation that we may choose to follow. If we decide based on our desires, we still need to be prepared to protect ourselves from unwanted pregnancy or disease and must also realize that sex can have an emotional impact on us.

Sex can bring up complicated feelings and emotions, not just about the person we're sharing it with, but about ourselves. Having sex might get wrapped up with our sense of self-worth or become the only way we feel it's possible to be intimate with someone. What's the motive for having any kind of sex when we don't totally want to? Is it to get love or attention or because we feel we have to? If we are not clearly choosing sex for ourselves, the experience may disturb us later.

Romance Novels: The Only Place Where Sex Is Always Perfect

His whole skin drank thirstily of her and when he thrust into her, he knew he had arrived at last at the source, the spring. Now, Daisy lay quietly, invaded, filled, utterly willing. She felt as if she were floating down a clean, clear river with birds singing in the trees on the bank. But there was more, more than this blissful peace, and together they quickened, panted, quested as eagerly as two huntsmen after an elusive prey, plunging through the forests of each other until they came at last to their victories, Daisy with a sound that was at least as much a cry of astonishment as it was of joy. She had experienced fulfillment before, but never with this excellence, this plenitude.
—Judith Krantz, *Princess Daisy*

Yikes! You have got to be kidding. We can get the most bizarre ideas about what sex should be like from the media. In romance novels, like the above bestseller, sex is often described as an awakening or an explosive event, far from what most of us experience in real life. Compared to romance novels, our own experiences may seem awkward or incomplete. Exploring our own sexuality is not about living up to some imaginary standard, but about enjoying our very real experiences.

To discover our own feelings and to make our own choices about being sexual—with our eyes open—it helps to hear other girls' feelings and experiences on the topic. In the following stories, girls share details of their first experiences, including how it did or did not change them, how they felt afterward, and things they'd just like other girls to know.

True Tales of First-Time Experiences

After the first time I had intercourse, I went into the bathroom and looked in the mirror expecting to see how grown up I was.

I was feeling very happy, and I looked back to the other room at the boy I had just lost my virginity to, and he was putting his retainer back in his mouth. My illusion of maturity was totally shattered. Back to reality.

—Camille, eighteen years old

My first time was fabulous.

I can't even explain it. He was my boyfriend for a year and a half. Sex to me is not just the physical side; it is more the emotional bond. Even though we are not going out anymore, I still love him.

—Rochelle, fifteen years old

"Losing" our virginity: Why is our first experience with intercourse a loss of anything? Why isn't it seen as a gaining of knowledge or experience? And why is there so much emphasis on the first time? It is supposed to be special—a "perfect" exchange with our true love and full of romance. In the real world, our first experiences with sex come in many shapes and forms. Sometimes the experience is wonderful and a cherished memory. Sometimes the first time is just not a big deal. Other times there is disappointment, especially when we have been building it into such a special occasion. If the first time is disappointing, there's room for improvement down the road.

After sex, I feel like I have opened myself up as much as I possibly can, being so close to another person.

I had sex for the first time this year. A lot of people said it was going to hurt so much the first time, but it didn't hurt at all. I wasn't in love with him, but we were friends. There was pressure, for me to have sex, mostly from my friends who had all had sex at fourteen, fifteen, or sixteen. It wasn't the kind of peer pressure like, "You have to do it," but I just felt like it was time. I told him I was a virgin because I thought it was important for me to communicate that. We went out for two weeks after that and then broke up.

People say wait until you're in love. I say, just don't do it when you're drunk or on drugs. At parties, some people get drunk and go to another room. I don't think that is the way to do it, you should be mature. At thirteen, you might not know it's more than sex you're getting into: like pregnancy and dealing with your feelings for the other person. At times my feelings change for the other person after sex, and I feel closer or farther apart. After sex, I feel like I have opened myself up as much as I possibly can, being so close to another person. It's lucky when you can find sex and close emotions together in a relationship.

—Margot, sixteen years old

I had done something major that I had never done before.

The first time I had sex was when I was in the eighth grade and had just turned thirteen. My boyfriend was sixteen and we had been dating for six months. I can't remember him asking me to have sex or me asking him—we just sort of did it. I didn't bleed, and it wasn't painful. We used condoms, but we didn't talk about it. He had a bunk bed, and the condoms were hidden behind magazine posters on the ceiling— totally convenient, but nowhere to be seen.

I got a little more attached to my boyfriend after we started having sex, but not because the sex was thrilling or orgasmic. What I liked most was the intimacy with him: no clothes, skin on skin, an intimacy I had never felt with him or anyone else before. I had sex a lot with him, and I was more romantic and more involved with him, but we broke up at the end of the summer.

After having sex, I felt like a real woman. I had done something major that I had never done before. I felt different because of what society tells us about sex. Nothing was happening to my body: No physical maturity sprouted once I had sex, it continued to take time.

—Yolanda, sixteen years old

I had waited so long because I wanted the time and place to be right.

It was last year. I was really old compared to my friends. I had been dating him for two years in high school. He was a year older and went to college my senior year. The first time I visited him, it happened. I sort of wanted to get rid of my virginity. I wanted to say, "Take it!" I felt like a leper because I was a virgin. I thought I was going to be more mature after sex, but actually I got depressed. After we had sex we didn't talk about it, and we stopped speaking after that. He just wanted sex and then "good-bye." I had waited so long because I wanted the time and place to be right. I wanted to feel ready and not lose my virginity in the back seat of a car.

He didn't know I was a virgin. I didn't say anything because I didn't want him to have that power over me. I would feel like he had taken something away from me, and I was also worried that he would tell his friends, like he had done something so powerful. I was embarrassed because I bled and didn't even realize until afterwards and there was blood in my underwear. I told him I had my period because I didn't want him to know I was a virgin. After sex I thought, "That's it?" It only hurt briefly, and then it was like, "La dee dah."

—Tina, eighteen years old

We trusted each other, which helped, and we were both totally comfortable with the fact that we were two females, but we kind of rushed.

My first time was last year. It was with a woman I was good friends with since the age of eleven. We met at a summer camp, and we saw each other every summer. She is a year older, and in the fall of her freshman year, I went to visit her in college. I knew something was going to happen. She asked, "Where do you want to sleep?" and I said, "I'll just sleep in your bed." We fooled around. For both of us it was our first experience with a girl. We trusted each other, which helped, and we were both totally comfortable with the fact that we were two females, but we kind of rushed. I stayed there five nights, and we had sex every night. By the end it was strange because having sex almost felt like an obligation. Part of it was we had a more emotional than physical relationship. She didn't write to me for a month after, and I thought it had to do with sleeping together. Sex does change things.

Having sex with her was a big relief for me. I almost always knew that I was bisexual, but I thought, "How can I really know I'm bi if I've never been with a woman?" I didn't know where I stood on the whole issue. Fooling around with her made me feel good, and more clear. I was proud.

—Angie, seventeen years old

Virgin Voyage

I'm a normal person who hasn't had sex, so abstinence is not impossible.

I have a boyfriend who understands why I don't want to have sex. I don't want to risk getting pregnant at all. I don't believe in abortion, so that is not an option for me. Having a baby right now would be impossible to manage. For these reasons, I want to be married before I have sex.

—Jessica, eighteen years old

It's easy to forget that our virginity does not determine our personality. We are all virgins at one time, and virgins can be cool, aggressive, clever, or nasty, just like anybody else. Lots of girls are virgins simply because they haven't found the right circumstances for sex yet. And that's cool, because it's great to wait rather than dive into an uncomfortable situation that we're not ready for. Some girls choose to abstain from sex and draw value and strength from such a decisive choice.

This may seem obvious, but remaining a virgin does not mean you are not a sexual being. Discovering our sexuality is a voyage—and it's not all about having sex. Our sexuality is shaped by the books and magazines we read, the movies we watch, the music we listen to, and the conversations we have. Sometimes we are exposed to new thoughts or descriptions of sexuality that bring a tingle to our toes or make us a lot more interested in the topic. Other times we might see or hear something that we find scary, alarming, or offensive. All of these experiences are part of our sexuality, it's not just about "doin' it" or "not doin' it." Positive sexual experiences are the ones that make us swoon and feel aroused. Maybe your feet are your favorite erogenous zone. Perhaps when your lab partner brushes your shoulder, you quiver. Maybe when a guy comments on how hot last month's *Playboy* centerfold was, you feel turned off. Remember, when it comes to your sexuality, you're in the driver's seat.

There's this whole idea that sex is the only sexy thing you can do.

As if holding hands isn't sexy or interesting. In the movies, actors holding hands certainly don't look interesting. The message in movies is: Unless there are lots of obstacles, why not have sex? So in that way there's pressure, just because sex is viewed as the thing to do.

—Valerie, seventeen years old

There is so much to do with just fooling around; you don't have to have sex.

I'm a virgin. I've been raised in such a way that I see sex is for marriage. There is such a stigma attached to sex in my religion. I used to not be comfortable with doing anything sexual; I would feel guilty. It wasn't until my senior year that I started touching boys in any way. Kissing and having boys feel my chest took me a long time. I'm so emotional, even just touching each other I worry, "Do we like each other enough?"

There is so much to do with just fooling around; you don't have to have sex. I do not want to deal with diseases or the possibility of getting pregnant. I also think sex should be saved for the one person you love. You should wait until you are more mature because you don't want to cry the next day. It's something you can't go back on. You can only do it once, so it should be when you know you'll never regret it.

—Miriam, nineteen years old

I value being a virgin, and I value that in other people, but I also appreciate the sexual experiences that I've had.

There are definitely groups where it is not cool to be a virgin. Just like in some groups it's cool to drink or do drugs. That's the "experienced woman of the world" group. The bad thing in that group is that if you're seventeen and eighteen and you haven't done that stuff, then it's like, "What's wrong with her, does she think virginity is so precious?" They call you "pure little goodie two shoes"—all that contempt. Second, there are groups where people try to be low-key about sex. They don't make a big deal about being a virgin or not being a virgin. That's the "we are way casual and cool" group. Last, there are groups where people pretty much don't consider

Let's Talk About Sex

It's easy to be confused by all the mixed messages about sex. Here are some books to help us sort things out for ourselves:

Am I the Last Virgin?: Ten African American Reflections on Sex & Love, edited by Tara Roberts, New York: Simon & Schuster, 1997.

Changing Bodies, Changing Lives: A Book for Teens on Sex and Relationships by Ruth Bell, New York: Times Books, 1998.

Dilemmas of Desire: Teenage Girls Talk about Sexuality by Deborah L. Tolman, Cambridge, MA: Harvard University Press, 2002.

How Sex Works: A Clear, Comprehensive Guide for Teenagers to Emotional, Physical, and Sexual Maturity by Elizabeth Fenwick, New York: Dorling Kindersley, 1994.

The Underground Guide to Teenage Sexuality: An Essential Handbook for Today's Teens and Parents by Michael J. Basso, Minneapolis: Fairview Press, 2003.

What Your Mother Never Told You about S-E-X by Hilda Hutcherson, New York: Putnam Books, 2002.

having sex, they're like, "Of course you're a virgin." If you're not a virgin, it's very hard to be close friends with them. I know because I used to be one of them. I don't know what I am now. I value being a virgin, and I value that in other people, but I also appreciate the sexual experiences that I've had. I feel like when I do have sex, it won't be a loss.

—Rebecca, seventeen years old

Reputations: Sluts vs. Studs (Don't You Talk to Me That Way!)

It seems like reputations are always the girls' responsibility.

If a girl sleeps around, you would say, "She's with a new guy every week, what is she doing?" If a girl dates a guy who had a new girl every week, you would say, "What is she thinking? He's with someone new all the time." So the bad reputation is always put on the girl. That's how I look at it too.

—Gilda, seventeen years old

In my school, reputations spread like wildfire.

There are some people who call girls "sluts," but it has more to do with what a girl is wearing than who she is sleeping with. A girl can be a virgin and wear a skimpy outfit and be called a slut. Guys are called "dumb jocks" or "airheads," but it has nothing to do with sex. Guys don't get reputations the way girls do.

—Hannah, fifteen years old

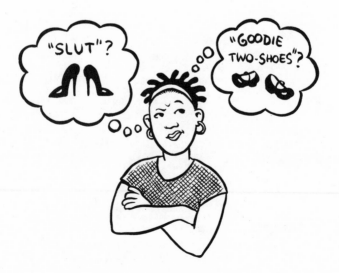

Here are some common contradictions we've come across:

"She's such a slut; she'll sleep with anyone."
"What a priss, waiting until she gets married."

"Oh gross, I can't believe you'd do that."
"What's your problem? Everyone's doing it."

"Masturbation is disgusting."
"You haven't experienced anything until you've had an orgasm."

"She dresses like she wants everyone to know she's easy."
"She's so boring; she dresses with a shirt buttoned up under her chin."

Guys are sometimes viewed as sleazy if they sleep around, but they are most often seen as studs. When girls are known for having lots of sex, we are often called sluts or described as promiscuous. Being called a slut may actually have nothing to do with our sexual activity: It may be because of our clothing or outgoing personality, or even jealousy on another person's part. But, whatever the reason, this label can taint a girl more than "sleazy" would taint a boy. The double standard is frustrating. With internet postings, instant messaging, and cell phone text forwarding, the slut label can be cruelly and quickly spread to larger audiences than the old fashioned anonymous scrawls on the bathroom stall.

Don't put up with other people's malicious labels. If we are called a slut or gossiped about, we should know that it is the other person who is not able to deal with their own baggage and ignorance. We should also make a point of not engaging in this "mean girl" behavior by refusing to pass on gossip or by supporting a girl who is not there to defend herself. As long as we show respect for ourselves and our partners, we can do whatever we are comfortable with, and no one else has the right to judge us. It's easier to ignore other people's opinions of our behavior if we are clear and sure in our decision making.

I tend to think I'm an exception to the female role in terms of sexuality.

I view sex as a notch on my belt and don't have a problem picking up a guy. Sex is an experience for me, and I don't have to be in love. The TV and the media rarely show women as that outgoing, unless they're evil characters. I find that when I initiate sex, it can scare guys. But if the guy's not ready, then I can take on the role of "Hey, that's cool" and pick up whatever we were doing and not go any further.

—Mariah, seventeen years old

Pressure: When the Heat Is On

He wasn't sensitive to the fact that I wasn't ready.

My sophomore-year boyfriend was pressuring me to have sex before I was ready to. He would say things like, "Come on, your mom will be out of town," even though I kept saying no. At school, he would also motion to me in a way that meant he wanted to have sex. I got the feeling he would have sex with anybody, it didn't matter who it was. I just happened to be in his life at the time. Even on the way to gym, he'd signal to me. He wasn't sensitive to the fact that I wasn't ready. I never had sex with him, but he made me feel bad about it.

—Camille, eighteen years old

It was lack of self-esteem on my part. I should have trusted my own feelings.

I had just started dating this guy, and he wanted to have sex. I said, "I don't want to have sex, it's just the beginning." He asked why and got all whiny. The next night we fooled around, and he brought up sex again as if we hadn't just talked about it the night before. He obviously wasn't listening to me and didn't care about what I wanted. I ended up having sex, but after that night I refused to date him again. He called several times, but I didn't want to see him. I told him, "You just don't get it." When I look back, it was as much my responsibility as his. It would have been easy for me to get up and walk away: He was small and scrawny, he couldn't have held me down. And he had roommates in the other room. I guess it was lack of self-esteem on my part. I should have trusted my own feelings, but instead I was like, "Oh well, I'll do it."

—Karina, eighteen years old

Deciding to have sex is complicated enough; the last thing we want to deal with is someone pressuring us. Unfortunately, many of us experience pressure—either from others or from ourselves. It may be someone insisting on intercourse as proof of our feelings ("but don't you love me?"), wanting unprotected sex ("but it feels better without a condom"), or asking us to do a sexual act we are not comfortable with ("but everyone else does that"). We can have sex when we want to, and if someone else can't respect that, they can just hit the road. We don't have to put up with someone whining at us to have sex or feel like we have to do something just to fit in.

Myth: If a date pays for my dinner, he has the right to expect something in return.
Reality: If he expects anything, it might be money for half the bill. We are never obligated to have sex or perform sexual favors.

Myth: Guys "need" to have sex more than women do. They feel terrible and can even get "blue balls" if they get an erection and don't have an orgasm, so we'd better do something to satisfy them.
Reality: We can feel the desire to have sexual fulfillment just as strongly as guys. And, a guy will not injure himself from not having sex! Not having an orgasm may be disappointing for a guy, but no more than it is for us to stop in the middle of sexual activity when we are turned on. Whenever we feel uncomfortable, we have the right to say so and stop.

Pressure, to me, is when a guy wants to have sex and I don't.

If a guy pressures me, I say, "Get out." I have no qualms. I try not to get myself in difficult situations. I have friends who will put themselves in situations that can be harmful, like being alone with someone they don't know that well. I like to be friends first with the people I date. A friend listens if I say no.

—Liz, eighteen years old

I was the last one of my friends to lose my virginity, and I gave in because of the pressure.

I was sixteen and didn't want to have sex at all, but I felt pressured into it by my boyfriend and my friends. I was sexually molested when I was younger, and my boyfriend knew this. He said I had to get over it and deal with it by having sex. Later, I realized that my boyfriend was really immature and a jerk to say I should have sex with him to get over being sexually molested. What actually helped me get through the pain of sexual abuse was not having sex, but talking about my past with friends who were supportive.

—Mica, eighteen years old

There have been moments in my life when I've felt pressure to have sex.
Other times I feel pressured to be less physically intimate than I want to.
Friends don't say, "You shouldn't be doing that," but I just feel like they wouldn't
approve. My friends don't pass a lot of judgments, but I still feel judged, just by the
fact that they aren't doing it. Other times I've felt pressure to have sex from the
world, from society. On my own, I feel pretty flexible about sex. I don't feel set
against it or set for it.

—Evelyn, sixteen years old

Lesbians and Bisexuals: It's Not Taboo

I kissed a girl
Her lips were sweet
She was just like kissing me
Kissing a girl won't change the world
But I'm so glad I kissed a girl

—Jill Sobule, "I Kissed a Girl," *Jill Sobule*

Being gay has always been a part of me.
My boyfriend from the sixth grade called me up three years after I started going out
with a female. He asked, "What happened to you? Why did you switch on me? What did
I do wrong?" I told him being gay wasn't in the drinking water, it wasn't in my bagel, it
wasn't in anything. Being gay has always been a part of me, whether or not I admitted
it at one time or another. He pretended he got it, but I don't think he understood.

—Layla, fifteen years old

Science may never be able to prove definitively what makes people attracted to each
other. Biological traits, early experiences, and environment may all play a part in
forming our sexual identity. Some girls say, "I always knew I was gay." Others say
their sexual identity became clearer as they got older. Still others find that using a
label, like lesbian or straight, is a problem because of the wide range of sexual feelings and experiences we all have. We may not choose to use a label for ourselves, but
instead take a stand outside of society's need to place us in neat categories. Or we
may choose to define our sexual orientation: that we are mostly attracted to men,
mostly attracted to women, or attracted to both genders. For many of us, identify-
ing as lesbian or bisexual is an essential part of expressing our sexuality.

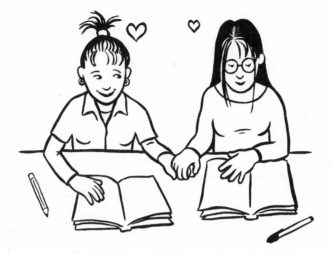

If you kiss a girl, it doesn't mean you're a lesbian necessarily.

I consider myself straight, but growing up I was always affectionate with my girlfriends. My best friend and I used to kiss in private. I enjoyed that and never thought about it in terms of my sexual identity.

—Meg, sixteen years old

You can't figure out if you are homosexual just by having a sexual experience.

There is this "straight until proven otherwise" thing. You can't call yourself gay until you've had a gay sexual encounter. Well, what if you haven't had sex at all? I knew I was gay before I ever kissed anyone. I had a friend who was questioning her sexuality. One day she asked me, "Will you have sex with me?" I said, "Why in the world do you want me to have sex with you?" She told me she was trying to figure out if she was gay or not. I said, "Do you honestly think that it works that way? If you like it, then you are, and if you don't, then you're straight?" You can't figure out if you are homosexual just by having a sexual experience.

—Kyra, eighteen years old

People think that if you're bisexual then you're confused.

I don't label myself. I think that labels serve to make other people comfortable, and I feel no need to do that. I'm pretty open about my sexuality to people, and most of my friends at school know I'm not straight. I've never lied about it. People think that if you're bisexual then you're confused and can't choose, and if you're *homosexual then you're obviously this radical. I feel no need to say I'm bisexual or homosexual. Even the gay community tries to define you. People feel better when they define someone else because they feel insecure themselves. I think when people try to get me to define myself, they feel uncomfortable more than anything else.*

—Carla, seventeen years old

Coming Out: A Lifelong Process

Coming out is often thought of as a one-time deal, but actually it is a lifelong process because we are constantly meeting people who do not know what our sexual orientations are. During our teen years, we are exploring sexual experiences—in a sense, trying them on. We are deciding what—and whom—we like sexually. This can be an exciting time, but also a confusing one, especially if we have sexual feelings for other girls. Though one in ten Americans considers himself or herself homosexual, our society emphasizes a heterosexual point of view. To be gay is like being "crooked" in a straight world. Everything from television shows to movies, songs, advertisements, and textbooks assumes we are attracted to people of the opposite sex.

Coming out to people can be frightening because it is unclear how people are going to react. Often, telling close friends or a family member is a relief because it lets them in on an important part of who we are.

I came out to my mom by leaving a poem on the kitchen table about a girl I liked.

My mom said, "I guess you are bisexual or something." I said, "Yeah, I don't think too much about it," which wasn't totally true. "Don't you think it would be easier if you picked gay or straight?" I told her, "Mom, I can't change the way I am." She ended with, "I want to make things easier for you." She was supportive. It was important to tell my mom and friends because both honesty and friendship are important to me.

I don't think anyone can really care for me if they don't know everything about me. I first told my close friends, who I knew I could tell anything to and not shock them. It was great because it wasn't a big deal to them. My friends are cool about it; they will sleep in the same bed with me and know it's not necessarily sexual at all.

—Angie, seventeen years old

The Kinsey Scale:
The Fluid State of Sexuality

Though labels can be helpful when categorizing individuals, many people are uncomfortable with being labeled or categorized when it comes to their sexual orientation. Rather than dividing our sexuality into strict categories—lesbian, straight, and bisexual—perhaps sexual orientation should be viewed as a natural continuum. In other words, our sexuality is a fluid spectrum, not an either/or situation. The Kinsey scale is based on a large study of male sexual behavior and, later, of female sexual behavior (yes, we count too!).[1] The scale depicts sexuality as a range of possibilities, a range in which very few people are 100 percent straight or 100 percent gay. Our sexual preferences may shift over time, by circumstance or by choice. The point of the scale is not to rate ourselves, but to realize the range of feelings we can have.

```
0_____1_____2_____3_____4_____5_____6
```

0   Heterosexual: never responds sexually, either emotionally or physically, to persons of the same sex

1   Heterosexual, with occasional attraction to persons of the same sex

2   Mostly heterosexual, with more than occasional attraction to persons of the same sex

3   Bisexual: equally attracted to persons of both sexes

4   Mostly homosexual, with more than occasional attraction to the opposite sex

5   Homosexual, with occasional attraction to persons of the opposite sex

6   Homosexual: never responds sexually, either emotionally or physically, to persons of the opposite sex.

Note: Check out the 2004 movie *Kinsey*, written and directed by Bill Condon, which depicts Dr. Kinsey's life and groundbreaking research.

Out and About

One out of every ten of us may be gay. The following will offer support as we discover our own sexuality:

Nonfiction Reading

Becoming Visible: A Reader in Gay and Lesbian History for High School and College Students edited by Kevin Jennings, Los Angeles: Alyson Publications, 1994.

Bi Any Other Name: Bisexual People Speak Out edited by Loraine Hutchins and Lani Kaahumanu, Los Angeles: Alyson Publications, 1991.

Different Daughters: A Book by Mothers of Lesbians edited by Louise Rafkin, San Francisco: Cleis Press, 2001.

Free Your Mind: The Book for Gay, Lesbian, and Bisexual Youth—and Their Allies by Ellen Bass and Kate Kaufman, New York: HarperPerrenial, 1996.

Generation Q: Gays, Lesbians, and Bisexuals Born Around 1969's Stonewall Riots Tell Their Stories of Growing Up in the Age of Information edited by Robin Bernstein and Seth Clark Silberman, Los Angeles: Alyson Publications, 1996.

The Lesbian Almanac compiled by The National Museum and Archive of Lesbian and Gay History, New York: Berkley Books, 1996.

Odd Girls and Twilight Lovers: A History of Lesbian Life in Twentieth-Century America by Lillian Faderman, New York: Columbia University Press, 1991.

Two Teenagers in Twenty: Writings by Gay and Lesbian Youth edited by Ann Herron, Los Angeles: Alyson Publications, 1994.

A Woman Like That: Lesbian and Bisexual Writers Tell Their Coming Out Stories edited by Joan Larkin, New York: Perennial, 2000.

Literature

Aimee and Jaguar: A Love Story, Berlin 1943 by Erica Fischer, Los Angeles: Alyson Publications, 1998.

Alma Rose by Edith Forbes, Seattle: Seal Press, 1993.

Annie on My Mind by Nancy Garden, New York: Farrar, Straus & Giroux, 1992.

Girls, Visions, and Everything by Sarah Schulman, Seattle: Seal Press,1986.

Good Moon Rising by Nancy Garden, New York: Farrar, Straus & Giroux, 1996.

Oranges Are Not the Only Fruit by Jeanette Winterson, New York: Atlantic Monthly,1998.

Patience and Sarah by Isabel Miller, New York: Fawcett Books, 1994.

Red Azalea by Anchee Min, New York: Pantheon Books, 1994.

Rubyfruit Jungle by Rita Mae Brown, New York: Bantam Books,1988.

Stone Butch Blues by Leslie Feinberg, Los Angeles: Alyson Publications, 2003.

Movies and Television Shows

Antonia's Line directed by Marleen Gorris, 1995. This quirky story chronicles four generations of women in a matriarchal family.

But I'm a Cheerleader directed by Jamie Babbit, 1999. This is a campy film about a young cheerleader who is sent to a reform school by her family hoping it will "straighten her out."

Go Fish directed by Rose Troche, 1994. *Go Fish* takes a sassy, playful look at love among a small circle of young lesbians.

The Incredibly True Adventures of Two Girls in Love directed by Maria Maggenti, 1995. Two teenagers unexpectedly experience first love.

The L Word directed by Lisa Cholodenko et al., 2004. This cable TV show portrays the lives and loves of a group of lesbian friends living in Los Angeles.

The Watermelon Woman directed by Cheryl Dunye, 1997. The search for the 1930s film actress known only as the Watermelon Woman is the impetus of this autobiographical film.

When Night Is Falling directed by Patricia Rozema, 1995. This visually stunning film is about a teacher at a religious school whose life is transformed when she falls in love with a circus performer.

It was almost a rebirth when I came out at school after accepting it myself.

When I was fifteen, in my sophomore year, I told my friends that I was gay. Part of me knew I was gay, but part of me was thinking, "I can say it, but it doesn't have to be true." It was almost a rebirth when I came out at school after accepting it myself. I don't think I could bear to not be "out" because there would be such a conflict between what I was feeling and what I was saying, or even not saying, and what I was doing.

I came out to my mother, and that was a really bad scene. She started crying. She said if she had brought me up differently I would have been straight. I told her, "Maybe I don't want to be straight. Maybe if I could go back and do it over again, I would decide to do the same thing." But when she met a girl in my dorm I had a relationship with, she was fine about it. She had been worried I was abnormal, but when she was introduced to a real person, it was okay and she could ignore the gender.

I don't know if I would have come out if I wasn't in a high school with lots of accepting people, partly because I wouldn't have felt safe. I wouldn't have the support of my friends or other role models to go by. I think I would have spent a lot more time alone rather than subjecting myself to social situations where I wouldn't have fit in. My advice to young lesbians in that position is, hang on and don't despair. There are other lesbians and bisexuals out there. Certainly high school is not forever, and you can choose to go to a college where there is a social scene where you fit in.

—Kyra, eighteen years old

I think it would have been a lot harder to come out if I was a guy.

I've noticed that when I tell male friends I'm gay, they often respond with, "Wow." They seem to get off on it, which is kind of disturbing. If a guy told them he was gay, they would probably freak out. From my experience, people think it's more of a natural thing for females to be physical with each other. Females have more cuddly friendships, and it's not such a huge step to kissing or whatever. Whereas for guys, one of the only times to be physical is during a football game when they slap each other on the backside.

—Wenji, seventeen years old

Homophobia: Fear of Queers

In ninth grade at a school dance, two girls kissed. I thought it was cool.

I was sure I was gay a year before my first lesbian experience. I had suspicions all my life, but I always thought, "No, anything but being gay." I had the feeling that being gay was perverse. I grew up in suburbia, where if you are gay you are an out-

cast. I felt, "How horrible—you can't have a husband and a kid." Starting in sixth grade I just wanted to fit in, but I'd have dreams of having sex with my best friend; I'd wake up and feel like I was a terrible creature.

In ninth grade at a school dance, two girls kissed. I thought it was cool. The next day everyone was talking about it saying, "That was disgusting." I wanted to say to them, "Shut up. You like me, and I think about doing that." But I didn't feel like I could tell anyone because they would think I was disgusting too. The jocks in my high school thought that being bisexual or gay was gross; if you expressed anything different, people would say, "Hey, what's the matter with you?" It's hard because our society can make you feel there must be something wrong with you if you don't make fun of gays.

—Leah, seventeen years old

These days, more people are publicly talking about gay viewpoints. And realistic gay characters are showing up in television shows, movies, and books. However, being gay is still treated as outside of what is "normal," and homophobia—the unreasonable fear or hatred of gays—is still common. Gay bashing—both psychological and physical—is unfortunately a reality at some high schools, and many students feel it is unsafe to come out in this hostile atmosphere.

Growing up as a bisexual or a lesbian in a world that considers you an exception can lead to strong feelings of isolation. Constantly receiving the message from society that we are not "normal" may partly explain why gay teenagers may be more likely to be suicidal than straight teenagers.[5] If we are lesbian or bisexual, reaching out to a gay community that feels pride in its identity can make us feel strong and not alone. Through a gay and lesbian hotline or a lesbian resource center, we can feel connected to a larger gay community.

If a resource center or hotline doesn't exist in your community, call the toll-free Gay and Lesbian National Hotline at (888) 843-4564, or go to www.glnh.org.

Some students are open-minded, but a lot are homophobic.

At my school, some students formed a gay club called "the ten percent club." Me and my friends were not concerned about it, we had the attitude that it's their business. But some of the girls in my homeroom decided they were going to form a straight club—an anti-gay club—because they felt there shouldn't be a gay club in our school. I said, "Wait a minute, they didn't form an anti-straight club. What is your problem? Why are you going to waste your energy on that?" I mean, these girls were spending forty

Vampire Lesbians and Other Incredible Tales

Historically, our culture has often ignored female homosexuality or labeled it as "school girls' nonsense." But when society has acknowledged lesbians, it has often done so with hatred or fear. In the past, lesbians have been described as evil, mentally ill, exotic, and even as vampires! Here's a glance at the portrayal of lesbians over the past centuries:

1800s Lesbianism gained a reputation for being abnormal, exotic, . . . and evil. In the 1800s, the science community categorized a "masculine" woman as being a man trapped inside a woman's body, leading to a lot of confusion about lesbians. In 1857, lesbians became associated with vampires in Charles Baudelaire's *Les Fleurs du Mal*, which includes poems that depict the lesbian as a mysterious monster who preys on her victims. (In the 1990s, gay writers reclaimed the vampire lesbian as a heroic archetype.)

1900–1950 In the first half of the 1900s, lesbians were still thought to be men born in women's bodies—members of the "third sex." Psychologists à la Freud chimed in, saying that early childhood trauma and penis envy can cause lesbianism. In the 1920s, lesbians became more visible, especially in artistic circles. But they were still portrayed as exotic and evil. The vampire image also endured, with the vampire usually described as beautiful, seductive, and destructive.

1950s–early 1960s In the ultimate era of nuclear-family Mom-and-Dadness, the lesbian was portrayed as a home and family wrecker, as in this 1954 quote from an old publication called *Jet*: "The lesbian, like the male homosexual, who stalks a married home has to be considered dangerous."[1] As if that weren't enough, she was considered lonely and twisted too!

Late 1960s Oh, the times they were a-changin'! Sister love became way cooler than in the fifties, and the lesbian feminist movement developed in the late sixties. Some extremists of the movement preached that if you were a feminist, you should choose to be a lesbian—creating a division among some women in the feminist movement.

1970s As the lesbian feminist movement blossomed, lesbians themselves began creating their own images of lesbian identity and sexuality. In books such as Rita Mae Brown's *Rubyfruit Jungle* (1973) sex between women is described as fulfilling—something to be enjoyed without any guilt.

1980s Radicals like Pat Califia fueled debates in the lesbian community by defending sadomasochism and reclaiming pornography for women. Diverse ways of being a lesbian or a bisexual were brought into the limelight.

1990s Being bisexual became "fashionable" for some women. Movies like *Chasing Amy* were enjoyed by more mainstream audiences. Ellen DeGeneres, the cool comedian, made waves (ranging from being called Ellen "Degenerate" to being celebrated as a heroine) as the first main character on a TV show to come out as lesbian.

2000s Lesbian chic creates an atmosphere of acceptance: We can now watch *The L Word* and a *Sex in the City* episode with Samantha dating a woman, or see pop icons kiss.

"Sure there's been progress, but it's not like the world is rallying around a burly dyke standing up for gay marriage"

—Steph, nineteen years old

There is still plenty of headway left to be made. Society, in general, has some room to grow in accepting lesbians who do not fit the heterosexual standard of being "pretty" or "hip."

minutes at lunch discussing how horrible it was to see two girls kissing in the hallway. They made it sound like it was the worst thing they ever saw. Some students are open-minded, but a lot are homophobic. They are like, "Don't do it near me."

—Destiny, sixteen years old

I feel like bisexuality and homosexuality are normal, and the kinds of cultures I respect all have gay acceptance integrated.

There's a clear atmosphere at my school of, "Yes, homosexuals need to be protected and accepted," but actually a lot of the acceptance is only on an intellectual level and not a physical and emotional level. Some people at school are uncomfortable with the concept and think being gay is pretty weird: "How do they do that?" "What do they do together?" But they've heard a lot about it politically and their families are liberal, so they're like, "Yes, we accept them."

I think it would be hard for a student to be gay at my school. Some people would become less physically affectionate to them and give them more room in the hall. Other people who were never their friends would come up and be friendly to them just because they were gay.

I feel like bisexuality and homosexuality are normal, and the kinds of cultures I respect all have gay acceptance integrated. In that way, I think I'm different from a lot of my friends.

—Rebecca, seventeen years old

Our headmaster said that he saw homosexuality as a lifestyle and a choice that has consequences.

He would tell us, "If you don't like how you are being treated, you should just choose not to be gay and that will solve your problem." I wonder about saying that to a straight person.

—Carla, seventeen years old

Myth: All lesbians want to sleep with me.
Reality: Gay women are not attracted to all women, just like straight women are not attracted to every man they see.

Myth: I have to fool around with a woman to know if I am a lesbian or bisexual.
Reality: It's possible to be a lesbian without ever having had a sexual encounter with a girl, in the same way a heterosexual girl doesn't need to kiss a boy to know she's straight.

Myth: What do lesbians do together? It must be really weird.

Reality: Lesbian lovers touch each other and don't do anything "weirder" than heterosexual lovers do together.

Myth: Having a crush on another girl is a sign of homosexuality.

Reality: Having crushes on other girls does not necessarily mean you are a lesbian. Many girls have fantasies or sexual experiences with other girls. Sexual preferences for a partner get more obvious as we get older.

Myth: A lesbian is a man trapped in a female body.

Reality: Lesbians are not men; they are women. A woman can look "masculine" and not be a lesbian, or can look "feminine" and not be straight.

Activism: Voicing Our Rights

At fourteen, I felt like an outcast because of my bisexual feelings.

I decided to be as different as possible. I joined the punk rock scene and became politically active. I went to gay marches, including the gay rights march in Washington, D.C. This helped a lot because most of the time I have had to hold back being bisexual, but there I could just relax. It's like having a back rub. Before, if I looked at a girl, I'd sort of slap myself and think, "Wait, do you know what she'd think if she knew?" But I realized that there are a lot more people who are gay than let on.

—Angie, seventeen years old

Gay activist groups are working nationwide to combat discrimination against gays and to make homosexuality more visible. The chant "We're here, we're queer, get used to it!" and the slogan Silence=Death are powerful statements about how important it is to be out, to show society that heterosexuals are not the only people on the planet. A current and very public battle that many people are fighting for is the right for gays to legally marry each other. But vocal and far-reaching activism is fairly recent.

Lesbians have been organizing since the early 1900s. The Society for Human Rights, established in Illinois in 1924, was the first homosexual activist organization. Sadly, it lasted only a few months, but it managed to produce two issues of the first publication on gay issues, *Friendship and Freedom*. In 1947, Lisa Ben started the

We're Here, We're Queer

"Queer" was originally used as a put-down for gays but has been reclaimed, starting with the activist group Queer Nation and its popular slogan: "We're here, we're queer, get used to it!" This organization was founded in 1990 and for a decade used direct action to create positive change for gay rights. Though the organization is not currently active, their embrace of the word "queer" lives on, as seen in the titles of gay supportive television shows (Queer Eye for the Straight Guy, Queer as Folk) and in its continued political use in gay communities.

Check out these organizations that champion queer rights and visibility:

AIDS Coalition to Unleash Power (Act-Up)

This activist group works for AIDS funding and research, in addition to queer visibility.
332 Bleeker Street, Suite G5, New York, NY 10014
email: actupny@panix.com
website: www.actupny.org

Gay and Lesbian Alliance Against Defamation

GLAAD is an organization dedicated to promoting and ensuring fair, accurate, and inclusive representation of people and events in the media as a means of eliminating homophobia and discrimination based on gender identity and sexual orientation.
5455 Wilshire Boulevard #1500, Los Angeles, CA 90036
phone: (323) 933-2240
248 W. 35th Street, 8th Floor, New York, NY 10001
phone: (212) 629-3322

Gay and Lesbian National Hotline

phone: (888) 843-4564
email: glaad@glaad.org
website: www.glaad.org

Human Rights Campaign

As America's largest gay and lesbian organization, this political group lobbies Congress to advance equality based on sexual orientation. It provides a national voice for lesbian, gay, bisexual, and transgender equal rights.

1640 Rhode Island Avenue NW, Washington, D.C. 20036

phone: (202) 628-4160

email: hrc@hrc.org

website: www.hrc.org

Indiana Youth Group

The hotline offers peer support to lesbian, gay, and bisexual youth. The website lists gay, lesbian, bisexual, transgender, and questioning youth groups (ages 13–24) in your area; it also offers peer-to-peer education.

hotline: (800) 347-TEEN

website: www.indianayouthgroup.org

Lesbian.org

This website promotes lesbian visibility on the internet and includes many links to areas of interest in politics, activism, arts, and culture.

website: www.lesbian.org

National Center for Lesbian Rights

NCLR is a national legal resource center with a primary commitment to advancing the rights and safety of lesbians and their families.

870 Market Street, Suite 370, San Francisco, CA 94102

phone: (415) 392-6257

email: info@nclrights.org

website: www.nclrights.org

National Gay and Lesbian Task Force

This group works to build the grassroots political power of the LGBT community in order to attain complete equality. It also helps attain pro-LGBT legislature.

1325 Massachusetts Avenue NW, Washington, D.C. 20036

phone: (202) 393-5177

(continued on next page)

(continued from previous page)

email: ngltf@ngltf.org
website: www.ngltf.org

Parents and Friends of Lesbians and Gays

This is a great support group for—you guessed it—the parents and friends
of lesbians and gays. They also work to fight homophobia. Check the phone
book for your local chapter, or call the national office in Washington, D.C.
1726 M. Street NW, Suite 400, Washington, D.C. 20009
phone: (202) 467-8180
email: info@pflag.org
website: www.pflag.org

Youth Resources

This website for lesbian and gay youth contains lots of personal stories, plus
great links to other queer youth websites.
website: www.youthresource.com

first lesbian magazine, *Vice Versa*. In 1955, Del Martin and Phyllis Lyon cofounded
Daughters of Bilitis, a lesbian group that in 1960 held the first national lesbian con-
ference in San Francisco.

However, it wasn't until 1969 that gay activism took off, when undercover police
raided the Stonewall Inn in New York City's Greenwich Village. The Inn was known
for its openly gay clientele, and the raid was an attempt to quash their sexual freedom. The gay community, tired of years of unjust treatment, rallied and fought back.
The Stonewall riot, as it is called, was a pivotal event in the gay community, leading
to the gay liberation movement. The Gay Liberation Federation was founded by
Stonewall participants as an ongoing militant political action group.

Today there are numerous gay rights and support groups (see the sidebar that
begins on page 146). These groups are great resources for activism as well as for
information and support. But we don't have to join a group or carry a sign to be
an activist for gay rights. Activism can mean writing a letter to your local repre-
sentative, marching in a parade, sharing a poem that expresses your sexuality,

standing up against others' homophobic comments, or coming out to an acquaintance. Any action we take that makes lesbians, gays, and bisexuals more visible is a form of activism.

Trusting Our Feelings

The more we can talk about our sexuality, the more powerful we can feel about it. With all the confused and mixed messages we get about sex and sexual orientation, the one thing we can always trust is our own feelings. We can't force ourselves to have experiences if we are not ready. If we're left feeling hurt, embarrassed, upset, uncomfortable, or burdened during or after sex, there's something wrong with what's going on. These kinds of feelings should be addressed, maybe with a friend, parent, or counselor. If we have been assaulted or abused, we need to seek information and guidance that will help us to heal and recover (more on this in the next chapter). Any kind of sex should leave us feeling mostly confident, happy, and satisfied. Getting together with others to talk about our experiences, ask questions, and share information helps us keep sexuality out in the open and in perspective.

6

Being in Charge of Our Sexuality

Protection: Being Informed and Safe

Once we've had the chance to decide how we want to explore our sexuality, we need to take responsibility for our decisions emotionally and physically. Knowing and following the facts about protection means saving ourselves from diseases and unwanted pregnancies. Whether we are sexually active or not, being informed is important. "Safer sex" means that we are using birth control to avoid pregnancy and sexually transmitted infections (STIs). Safer sex is also more than just knowing the facts—it's about making smart decisions and talking with our partners openly.

Most teens are responsible about having safer sex. Three out of four teens use protection—usually condoms—their first time,[1] and the majority continue using protection regularly after that.[2] This is an impressive statistic given that only half of all fifteen-year-olds say that their parents have talked to them about birth control or STIs.[3] Those who do not use protection are at serious risk for getting an STI or becoming pregnant. The reality is that if we're armed with the facts, being sexual can be healthy and enjoyable. If we choose to explore sexual intercourse or oral sex, we can inform ourselves first and use the best protection so that we are at extremely low risk for unwanted pregnancies or infections and can feel safe about what we are doing.

We used a condom.

Sex without a condom, to me, is not sex. It's just stupidity.

—Kimra, sixteen years old

151

I used to think that using a condom could ruin the moment.

This is really awful, and I'm so embarrassed about it, but the last three guys I had sex with, we didn't use a condom. Since I'm on the pill, pregnancy isn't an issue, and so I didn't bother to bring up the topic of condoms. I used to think that using a condom could ruin the moment. Afterwards I always worry about STIs and AIDS, and I think, "Damn, I should have used a condom." But I didn't, and that's the only thing that matters. This is dumb, but I think that a guy I'm with wouldn't have AIDS. Now I've made a pact with myself: The next guy I'm with will use a condom.

—Allie, seventeen years old

After that, he used a condom without a problem.

When we were about to have sex, he didn't bring up birth control. So I did. I said, "This is very important," and he didn't think it was. I was shocked. Can someone be that stupid not to use a condom? I pushed him away and said, "This isn't going to happen unless you use a condom." He said, "Okay. Diseases and stuff, I guess." He had a condom in his desk drawer. After that, he used a condom without a problem.

I can't imagine taking that risk. How can you not care? I have a close friend at school who was scared that she might be pregnant. Later I found out that she didn't use birth control. I was surprised. It ended up that she wasn't pregnant, but she still doesn't use protection. I think that's stupid. The consequences are so horrible that it is just not worth it.

—Barrette, seventeen years old

Barriers to Using Barriers

Each year, between 800,000 and 900,000 American girls age nineteen or younger become pregnant.[4] Each year, 20,000 young people are newly infected with HIV (the human immunodeficiency virus, which causes AIDS), and nearly four million new STI infections occur among fifteen- to nineteen-year-olds.[5] Despite these facts, there are still obstacles to getting information about safer sex. We don't see commercials on television advertising contraception because the networks are afraid they would be too controversial and "morally offensive" to their viewers. Our sex education classes may only teach, "If it's not yours, don't touch it." Some pharmacies keep the condoms in a case behind the cash register or don't sell them at all. Few middle school and high school students live in areas where their schools are allowed to give out condoms. So we might have to search on our own to find accurate information on birth control and the prevention of STIs. Family planning clinics, such as Planned Parenthood or your local women's health clinic, are great resources for free information about contraception and safer sex. See the sidebar on pages 158–159 for more resources.

Get the Facts

To be in control of our bodies, it's important that we know the truth about protection from STIs and pregnancy. There are many myths floating around; we need to get wise to the facts and not believe the myths that are wrong, wrong, WRONG. Here are a few popular ones:

Myth: If the guy pulls out I won't get pregnant because pre-come doesn't have sperm.

Reality: Pre-come does have sperm, and we can get pregnant and/or get an STI from it.

Myth: If I douche after sex, I won't get pregnant or get an STI.

Reality: Douching is used to eliminate vaginal odors; it is not designed and is not effective for preventing pregnancy or STIs.

Myth: I can't get pregnant the first time I have sex.

Reality: Yes, you can. When we are not using protection, we are putting ourselves at risk for pregnancy the first time we have sex, as well as the second time, the third time . . .

Myth: I can't get pregnant if I have sex during my period.

Reality: Sperm can live up to five days in a woman's body. The fact is, while we may be more likely to become pregnant mid-cycle, we have a chance of conceiving any time of the month.

Myth: I only fool around with other girls, so I don't have to worry about protection.

Reality: STIs may be passed from one girl to another through oral sex and through the exchange of vaginal fluids. Dental dams (see the section on contraception beginning on page 157) protect us from transmitting STIs during oral sex.

Myth: All condoms are like chain-link fences: They have tiny holes that allow the transmission of HIV.

Reality: Laboratory tests have shown that viruses, including HIV, cannot pass through latex or polyurethane condoms.[6] Lambskin condoms have been shown to be ineffective against HIV transmission, so we need to make sure the condom label says "latex" or "polyurethane." Unless it breaks or slips off, the right condom used properly prevents the transmission of HIV.

Why We Can Know the Facts and Still Not Protect Ourselves

Girl: "I'm sure he's going to pull out—he knows I'm unprotected."
Boy: "She must be on the pill—she hasn't asked me to use a condom."

We can be very intelligent, know the facts and have access to contraceptives but *still* not use them. According to one study, one-third of sexually active teenagers used contraception inconsistently and 31 percent reported that they were completely unprotected the last time they had sex.[7] Why is that? There seems to be more to safer sex than knowing the how's and why's of protecting ourselves. Sometimes, all

Fantasy Island: Where Sex Is Dreamy and You Don't Have to Worry About Protection

In the real world, sex is not something that just "happens." In reality, there are awkward moments, conversations about using protection, fears of catching diseases or getting pregnant, and fumbling with condoms. In the fantasy world created by television and movies, no one gets HIV or other STIs or gets pregnant, unless it's the central theme of the story.

The following is based on an actual scene from a popular TV series:

"Debbie" and "Dean" work together. They have flirted but never kissed. On this night, Dean arrives at Debbie's house and climbs the trellis to her window and wakes her. Debbie comes to the window in her bathrobe.
    DEAN: I have something I want to ask you.
    DEBBIE: Ssh. Try to be quiet. We don't want to wake my parents.
    DEAN: I'm sorry that I didn't know what I wanted before, but I know what I want now, and it's you.
    Debbie steps back to allow Dean to climb into her bedroom. Seductive music begins. She pulls off her robe, revealing a silky nightgown. He pulls off his jacket, and they begin to kiss. She removes his sweater, and he unbuttons his shirt. He fondles her hair and runs his hand down her arm. They continue

the education and correct information goes out the window in the heat of the moment. Planning ahead can make us stick to our decision to use protection.

There are many reasons people don't protect themselves. Here are some common ones:

- In the rush of passion, it's easy to believe, "Oh, it won't happen to me. I won't get pregnant or get an STI."
- It's too embarrassing to buy condoms or dental dams, or we're too shy to bring up their use with our partner.
- We're too cheap to buy contraceptives.

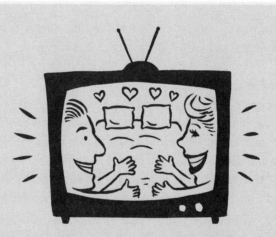

kissing with no words between them. She helps him take off his shirt. He lies back onto her bed. They continue kissing in perfectly choreographed movement. Lights fade. Music fades. Break to commercial.

What's missing from this picture? Yes, it's very sensual and romantic, but did they have sex? We're supposed to think so, but did they ever discuss it? Nope. And did they even mention birth control or protection from STIs? Nope again! To see any realistic sex scenes on television, we probably have to watch a PBS documentary on the mating habits of monkeys. Sure, it's fun to watch romance and melodramas—just keep the soap operas in perspective. Using a condom may not be as romantic as the smooth sex scenes on TV or in movies, but those are actors, and these are our lives.

- We're too drunk or high to remember to use birth control.
- Our partner doesn't want to use protection ("It doesn't feel as good with a condom"), and we go along with it.
- We think we want to have a baby.
- We think we don't need to use protection for oral sex because that is not "real" sex.

Choosing to have safer sex means deciding what to do about protection. Even the most effective methods of contraception won't work if used incorrectly. Thinking about protection but not following through in the actual moment will not help us. Protecting ourselves is not always easy or convenient: The condom may be in his jacket in the car while we are with Prince Charming in the forest. But if we don't drag ourselves back to the car to get the condom, we risk getting pregnant or contracting HIV or other STIs. We need to ask ourselves: Is it worth trading a moment of passion for consequences that can have a lifelong impact? It is our choice.

He didn't want to use condoms.

Six months ago, I had a serious boyfriend who was a lot older than I was. He didn't want to use condoms; he knew we should, but he didn't enjoy sex as much with them. Our relationship became serious fast, and we wanted to have sex. We talked about it and decided to use the rhythm method. Every time we had sex, it was like, "We're playing with fire." Not using birth control had to do with the relationship we had. I was romanticizing it because part of me wanted to find my "soul mate." I felt like a hypocrite because I've always been a huge supporter of birth control, and I was a peer counselor for AIDS awareness and did community outreach. So at the same time that I was having sex and not using condoms, I was aware of the risk. I kept thinking, "What's wrong with me?" My generation, the "safer sex" generation, grew up knowing about AIDS and condoms, and here I was not using one.

—Jackie, eighteen years old

I didn't care if I got pregnant because I was so in love with him.

When I was fifteen, we didn't use any contraception. I trusted him so much that I didn't care about protection. But that was a bad idea because trusting him wasn't what kept me from getting pregnant. I was ignorant. If I had gotten pregnant, I would have definitely had the baby. I didn't believe in abortion, and I wanted to marry him. I never got pregnant, which I'm very thankful for now.

—Sari, seventeen years old

Contraception: What, Where, and How

During a year of unprotected sex, we have an almost 90 percent chance of getting pregnant or contracting an STI. Effectively using contraception is essential for staying healthy and avoiding unwanted pregnancies. The following is a list of common contraceptives, intended to help us know what is available, how to get the most from these options, and what to watch out for. Rather than wait until the heat of the moment, we can do our shopping and practice using these methods ahead of time.

Male Condom

A thin cover worn over the penis during sexual intercourse and during anal and oral sex. It's called the "male" condom because it is worn by the boy, but it does not mean that we can't be in control in terms of having our own supply and being the one who knows how and when to use it. There are three types of male condoms: latex, polyurethane, and lambskin. To protect ourselves from STIs, we should use latex or polyurethane, as lambskin condoms are effective only for pregnancy prevention and don't prevent the transmission of HIV, hepatitis B, or the herpes simplex virus. To help prevent pregnancy, condoms should be used with a spermicide because this provides double coverage (and you can feel doubly safe just in case, in the rare event, the condom tears). Many condoms come prepackaged with spermicide (See more on spermicides on the next page). After one use, the male condom is discarded.

Where to get them: Condoms are the easiest and cheapest protection. They can be bought at most drugstores, supermarkets, online, and at some school or restroom vending machines. Sometimes they are kept behind the counter at pharmacies. We may feel embarrassed to ask the salesperson, but don't let a little bashful moment get in the way of protecting yourself. Condoms can also be found (often for free) at some student health centers and reproductive health clinics such as Planned Parenthood or our local women's health clinic.

Possible side effects: A small number of women are allergic to latex and experience vaginal irritation from using latex condoms. Polyurethane condoms are a good alternative if we have an allergy to latex.

Making Sex Safer

Being informed is the best way to make choices about sex. Here are some resources that provide information and answer questions:

Books

AIDS: What Teens Need to Know by Barbara Christie-Dever, Santa Barbara: Learning Works, 1996.

The Birth Control Book: A Complete Guide to Your Contraceptive Options by Samuel A. Pasquale and Jennifer Cadoff, New York: Ballantine, 1996.

GirlSource: A Book by and for Young Women about Relationships, Rights, Futures, Bodies, Minds, and Souls edited by GirlSource Inc., Berkeley, CA: Ten Speed Press, 2003.

The New Good Vibrations Guide to Sex by Cathy Winks and Anne Semans, San Francisco: Cleis Press, 2002.

Websites

Access to Voluntary and Safe Contraception
Information on contraception is provided at this website.
www.avsc.org

The Body
The Body provides information on the prevention, transmission, and treatment of HIV with resources from thirty top AIDS organizations across the country.
www.thebody.com/safesex

The Cafe Herpe
Sponsored by SmithKline and Beecham, Cafe Herpe provides information, support, and chats for young people with herpes.
www.cafeherpe.com

Coalition for Positive Sexuality: Sex Ed for Teens
Information on sexuality, safer sex, and decision-making for teens is what you'll find at this website.
www.positive.org

The following websites are designed to help answer your sexuality questions:

Ask Beth
www.ppsp.org/askbeth/askbeth.html

Go Ask Alice!
www.goaskalice.com

I Wanna Know (sponsored by the American Social Health Association)
www.iwannaknow.org

Scarleteen
www.scarleteen.com

SEX, etc. (a website for teens by teens)
www.sxetc.org

Teenwire (sponsored by Planned Parenthood)
www.teenwire.com

Hotlines
Toll-free (800) numbers are free and will not appear on your phone bill.

Emergency Contraception Hotline (800) 584-9911

Herpes Hotline (919) 361-8488

National AIDS Hotline (800) 342-AIDS

National AIDS Hotline in Spanish (800) 243-7889

National STD Hotline (800) 227-8922

Planned Parenthood Hotline (800) 230-PLAN

Note: Carrying a condom around for a long time in a pocket or wallet or exposing a condom to heat can damage or weaken the condom. Check the expiration date—if you are not sure of the condom's condition, throw it out. Condoms are the most commonly used form of birth control for first intercourse. Besides abstinence, condoms are the best protection against STIs that can be contracted from intercourse. Using *water*-based lubricants and spermicides with condoms can make sexual intercourse more enjoyable: a small drop inside the condom for the guys and some outside for us girls. Vaseline and any other oil-based products should never be used with latex condoms because they erode the material.

Everyone around knows I give importance to condoms.

There are one hundred condoms in my room. It's hard to escape them. It's a

How to Use a Condom

1. Before putting on the condom, the penis needs to be hard (erect).
2. Put the condom on the penis (either partner or both can do this) before the penis touches the vagina, mouth, or anus because pre-ejaculation fluid (pre-come) has sperm in it and can also carry diseases.
3. When putting the condom on, hold the tip of it to squeeze out the air and leave space for the semen.
4. Roll the condom all the way to the base of the penis. If you're having a hard time rolling it down, it may be inside out.
5. After sex, withdrawal needs to happen while his penis is still hard—so no semen leaks out. Hold the rim of the condom against the base of the penis as he slowly pulls out of your vagina.
6. Take the condom off carefully and throw it out—don't use it again. And congratulate yourself for having safer sex.

Condom Dos and Don'ts

DO use latex or polyurethane (plastic) condoms.

DO keep condoms in a cool, dry place.

joke among my friends. I am completely up front about the fact that I use condoms. Not that I would force my judgment on anyone else—I mean, that's their choice and this is my life.

—Angie, fifteen years old

Female Condom

This female counterpart to the male condom is a plastic baglike sheath made of polyurethane that fits inside the vagina. When used properly, this is the best method of protection against STIs after the male condom—giving females the option of an effective barrier method that they are in charge of wearing. Thin and strong, it is placed inside the vagina before intercourse and anchored by two flexible rings: one at the cervix and one outside the vagina. The ring at the closed end of the pouch is

DO put the condom on an erect (hard) penis before there is any contact with a partner's genitals.

DO use plenty of water-based lubricant (like K-Y Jelly or Astroglide) with latex condoms. This reduces friction and helps prevent the condom from tearing.

DO squeeze the air out of the tip of the condom when rolling it over the erect penis. This allows room for the semen (ejaculate, come).

DO hold the condom in place at the base of the penis before withdrawing (pulling out) after sex.

DON'T use out-of-date condoms. Check the expiration date carefully. Old condoms can be dry, brittle, or weakened and can break more easily.

DON'T unroll the condom before putting it on the erect penis.

DON'T use oil-based products, like baby or cooking oils, hand lotion, or petroleum jelly (like Vaseline) as lubricants with latex condoms. The oil quickly weakens latex and can cause condoms to break.

DON'T use a sharp object to tear open a condom wrapper. It's very easy to tear the condom inside. If you do tear a condom while opening the wrapper, throw that condom away and get a new one.

inserted into the vagina and adjusted so that it is against the cervix. The ring at the open end is kept outside of the vagina. The inside of the female condom is coated with a silicone lubricant, and once in place, the erect penis can slide into it for protected intercourse. Like the male condom, it is intended for one-time use.

Where to get them: Drugstores, online, or health clinics.

Possible side effects: We may have sensitivity to the silicone lubricant, and some people may experience insertion difficulties (practice always helps).

Dental Dam

A square piece of latex that covers the vagina, clitoris, and vulva for safe oral sex. Usually sold as six-inch by eight-inch sheets, they also come in flavors such as grape, mint, vanilla, strawberry, and banana.

Where to get them: Dental dams are available at some drug stores, online, from student health services, and at lesbian and gay community centers. Dentists also have them. If we can't find dental dams, we can buy latex gloves or condoms and cut them carefully into large pieces to put over the vagina and clitoris of our partner.

Possible side effects: A small number of women are allergic to latex.

Spermicide

Various forms (foams, jellies, creams, films, suppositories) of sperm-killing chemicals that are placed in the vagina before intercourse. They are most effective against pregnancy when used with a barrier method (condom, diaphragm, or cervical cap) and are considered ineffective in protecting us from STIs without a condom. Nonoxynol-9 is the most common chemical used in spermicides, and though at one point it was considered effective in preventing some STIs and HIV, we now know this is not true (see note below). Spermicide needs to be reapplied every time we have intercourse. Some spermicides give protection right away (like foam and gels), but the suppositories and films must be placed in the vagina at least fifteen minutes before sex so they have enough time to dissolve and spread. All forms of spermicides are effective when inserted less than one hour before intercourse. If *more* than one hour goes by before having sex, or if you have sex again, another application of spermicide is needed. Spermicide should not be washed or douched away for at least six hours *after* having sex.

Besides killing sperm, spermicide jellies and creams can serve as a lubricant, adding moisture to the vagina, which can make sex feel better. Lubricants that do not contain spermicides, however, offer no protection against STIs or pregnancy.

Some of us find the messiness of spermicides bothersome. Using a panty liner after having sex can help.

Where to get them: They may be purchased without a prescription at pharmacies and online. Some condoms already contain spermicides and are labeled, "spermicidal lubrication" or "spermicidal lubricant."

Possible side effects: Some of us feel burning or itching when we use spermicides. This is usually an allergic reaction. If we experiment with different brands, we may find one that does not irritate. If not, we need to find another method. Spermicides may also increase the risk of urinary tract infections.

Note: In the past, public health experts recommended using condoms combined with spermicides containing Nonoxynol-9 (N-9) for increased protection against HIV infection. Two recent studies, however, call into question the effectiveness and safety of N-9 because the chemical can irritate the vagina and increase the chances of an infection. Now, the Centers for Disease Control state that "N-9 should not be recommended as an effective means of HIV-prevention."[8]

Myth: Spermicides can make us infertile.

Reality: Spermicides have no effect on our future ability to get pregnant.

Diaphragm

A flexible, dome-shaped latex disk that keeps sperm from entering the uterus by holding spermicide in place against the cervix. It is palm-sized and covers the back of the vagina, including the cervix. Before having sex, spread about one to two teaspoons of spermicide on the inside of the diaphragm. Put the coated diaphragm inside the vagina, making sure the cervix is covered. We must insert it less than six hours before intercourse (though the closer to the time of intercourse, the better) and must leave it for *at least* six hours after intercourse (but not longer than twenty-four hours). If we have intercourse again within the six hours, spermicide must be added with an applicator (leaving the diaphragm in place).

Where to get one: A health care provider must fit us for a diaphragm. They will also show us how to use it (it takes practice). After a year of use, we should be refitted by a health care provider.

Possible side effects: May cause allergic reactions, urinary tract infections, and, in rare cases, toxic shock syndrome.

Note: We can't borrow a friend's diaphragm; they need to be fitted to us. This method's effectiveness is greatly reduced without spermicide.

Cervical Cap

A thimble-shaped, soft rubber cap that keeps sperm out of the uterus by forming a nearly airtight seal over the top of the cervix. Place a small amount of spermicide on the inside of the cap, and insert the cap into the vagina. The cap provides no protection without spermicide, which kills the sperm and strengthens the seal between the cap and the cervix. We can insert the cap up to twenty-four hours before intercourse, and we must leave it in for at least six hours after intercourse.

Where to get one: A health care provider must fit us for the cap and show us how to use it.

Possible side effects: May cause allergic reactions, increase your chance of a urinary tract infection, and, in rare cases, cause toxic shock syndrome. We should also have a regular pelvic exam to check for any inflammation around the cervix.

Note: We should not use the cervical cap during our period. We need to be refitted for the cap once a year.

FemCap

The FemCap is a silicone cup shaped like a hat with a groove between the dome and the brim. It includes a removal strap and fits securely in the vagina to cover the cervix. The FemCap comes in three sizes, determined by the inner diameter of the rim: small, for women who have never been pregnant; medium, for women who have had an abortion or a Cesarean delivery; and large, for women who have given birth vaginally. Like the diaphragm and cervical cap, it is used with spermicide. The FemCap can be worn for up to forty-eight hours at a time. Unlike the diaphragm and cervical cap, it is made from silicone, which is useful for women with sensitivity to latex. The FemCap is reusable for up to two years.

Where to get one: The FemCap is available only by prescription from a health care provider.

Possible side effects: We may have an allergy to the silicone or to the spermicides. Some women may forget and leave the FemCap in longer than forty-eight hours, increasing the chances of infection.

Lea Shield ("the Lea" or shield)

The Lea Shield is a soft, pliable cup made from silicone with an air valve and a loop for easy insertion and removal. The Lea prevents sperm from entering the cervix. It must be used with a spermicide and left in place for eight hours after sex to be effective. Like the diaphragm and the cap, the shield is inserted into the vagina before intercourse, is reusable up to six months, and is available only by prescription. Unlike the diaphragm and cap, it is one size fits all.

Where to get one: The Lea Shield is available only by prescription from a health care provider.

Possible side effects: We may have an allergy to the silicone or to the spermicides.

Contraceptive Sponge

The contraceptive sponge is a soft, disposable, disc-shaped device made from polyurethane foam that is inserted into the vagina and covers the cervix. The sponge is designed to absorb and trap sperm and contains spermicide. It has a string loop that helps with removal. Before inserting, the sponge is moistened with tap water to activate the spermicide, then gently squeezed until sudsy. It is placed into the

Which Contraceptive Methods Protect Us Against STIs?

- Polyurethane or latex condoms offer the fullest protection against STIs. Male and female condoms prevent contact with seminal and vaginal fluids during sex that involves penetration (anal, oral, or vaginal). Condoms aren't foolproof: You may be able to get genital herpes or warts because they can be located on the external genitals (where they are not covered by the condom).

- Diaphragms, cervical caps, the contraceptive sponge, and the Lea Shield give us some protection against STIs. These methods act as barriers for the cervix and the entry to the uterus but provide no protection for the inside of the vagina.

- Spermicides alone are *not* effective against STIs, meaning that condoms must always be used with spermicide to protect against STIs.

- The pill, Depo-Provera, the patch, the vaginal ring, and the IUD offer no protection against STIs. These methods are only effective for preventing pregnancy. To protect ourselves from STIs when using one of these devices, we should also use a condom.[1]

vagina with the dimple-side facing up and the string loop facing down. The cup-like indentation helps keep the sponge centered on your cervix.

The contraceptive sponge, or Today Sponge, was first introduced in 1983 and quickly grew in popularity due to its simplicity: it requires no prescription and can be kept in place up to twenty-four hours. However, the Today Sponge was taken off the market in 1994, when the Food and Drug Administration reported that it had found that water at the company's factory was contaminated. The current Today Sponge was reintroduced in 2003 and is produced by a different company (though it has kept the Today Sponge name).

Where to get it: We can purchase the contraceptive sponge online.

Possible side effects: Some of us find it difficult to remove the sponge, or we may forget to take it out all together (putting us at risk for an infection or, in rare cases, toxic shock syndrome). Some of us may also be allergic to the spermicide.

Oral Contraceptives (birth control pills, or "the pill")

Taken daily, oral contraceptives, which contain synthetic hormones, prevent pregnancy by keeping our ovaries from producing and releasing eggs and by thickening the cervical mucus to keep sperm from joining the egg. There are combination pills that contain estrogen and progestin and progestin-only pills (which are good for women who cannot take estrogen).

As the most effective contraception for pregnancy prevention (99.7 percent when used correctly[9]), it makes sense that the pill is used by more than one million teenage women (44 percent of all teenage women who use contraceptives[10]); however, oral contraceptives do not prevent STIs, and we must keep this in mind when playing it safe.

Where to get it: The pill requires a prescription from a doctor or health care provider.

Possible side effects: Nausea, weight gain or loss, puffiness, dark patches on the face (often a response to the estrogen in oral contraceptives), breast tenderness, breakthrough bleeding or spotting, loss of monthly period, vaginal infections, headaches, and mood changes. More serious but uncommon side effects include blood clots, heart attack, and high blood pressure.

Note: We must take the pill every day that it is prescribed at the same time of day for it to work. It does not protect against STIs. Some of us use the pill to regulate menstrual cycles or help with acne. Annual exams and Pap smears are especially important while using oral contraceptives. In addition, smoking while taking oral contraceptives is not recommended, as it increases our risk for a heart attack, breast cancer, blood clots, and strokes.[11]

Depo-Provera ("the shot")

Depo-Provera is a hormone (progestin) that is injected by a health care professional into a woman's buttocks or arm muscle every three months (pregnancy prevention begins twenty-four hours after injection). It prevents pregnancy in three ways: by inhibiting ovulation, by changing the cervical mucus to help prevent sperm from reaching the egg, and by changing the uterine lining, making it difficult for a pregnancy to occur. Depo-Provera does not protect us from STIs.

Where to get it: The shots are given by a doctor or at a health clinic.

Possible side effects: Weight gain, irregular periods, and bleeding between cycles.

Note: Although it has not been proven, some scientists believe that prolonged use of Depo-Provera may decrease bone mass in young women. You can reduce your risk of bone-mass loss by eating a healthy diet, taking calcium supplements, and getting regular weight-bearing exercise, like walking, running, and weight lifting.[12]

The Patch (Ortho-Evra)

The patch is a thin plastic patch that is placed on the skin of the buttocks, stomach, upper outer arm, or upper torso once a week for three weeks in a row. A new patch is worn each week, and the patch is not worn the fourth week, during menstruation. The patch protects against pregnancy by releasing estrogen and progestin to prevent ovulation (the release of the egg) and thickening cervical mucus to keep sperm from joining the egg.

The patch works best when it is changed on the same day of the week for three weeks in a row. Pregnancy can happen if an error is made in using the patch—especially if it becomes loose or falls off for more than twenty-four hours or the same patch is left on the skin for more than one week. With correct use, it is highly effective in preventing a pregnancy but ineffective in preventing STIs.

Where to get it: The patch requires a prescription from a doctor or health care provider.

Possible side effects: A skin reaction at the site of application. Results from long-term studies won't be available for some time, but researchers assume the disadvantages of using the patch are similar to the disadvantages of using the combination birth-control pill.[13]

Note: Don't smoke while you use the patch. Doing so may increase your risk of heart attack, blood clots, and stroke. The patch may not be as effective for women who weigh more than 198 pounds.

Vaginal Ring (NuvaRing)

The vaginal ring is a small, flexible ring, about two inches in diameter and an eighth of an inch thick, that is self-inserted deep into the vagina for three weeks in a row and then taken out during the fourth week for menstruation. Like the patch and the combination pill, the vaginal ring protects against pregnancy by releasing estrogen and progestin to prevent ovulation. It also thickens cervical mucus to keep sperm from joining the egg, and it may prevent a fertilized egg from implanting in the uterus.

Where to get it: The vaginal ring requires a prescription from a doctor or health care provider.

Possible side effects: Increased vaginal discharge, vaginal irritation, and infection. It may not be suitable for women who have weak pelvic muscles or chronic constipation. As with the patch, results from long-term studies won't be available for some time, but researchers assume the disadvantages of using the ring are similar to the disadvantages of using the combination pill.[14]

Intrauterine Contraceptive Device (IUCD or IUD)

An Intrauterine Device (IUD) is a small object that is inserted by a clinician through the cervix and placed in the uterus to prevent pregnancy. A small plastic string hangs down from the IUD into the upper part of the vagina. Once inserted, the IUD is effective immediately and may be kept in place for up to ten years (but we need to be checked periodically for signs of infection or in case of the rare possibility that the IUD has been expelled by the body). In general, as teenagers, we are not given IUDs as other safer methods are preferred. Also, the uterus of a young woman (who has not had a child) may be unable to hold an IUD.

No one knows exactly how the IUD really works, but experts think the IUD affects the way the sperm or egg moves, preventing fertilization. It also changes the lining of the uterus and prevents implantation. There are two types of IUDs available: ParaGard and Mirena. The ParaGard has a tiny copper wire wrapped around the plastic body and should not be used by anyone who is allergic to copper. The Mirena releases small amounts of a synthetic progesterone hormone, which helps to decrease the excessive bleeding and cramping that some women have with the IUD.

Where to get one: A medical exam is required to get an IUD, and a clinician must do the insertion.

Possible side effects: Heavy menstrual cycles, bleeding between periods, and abdominal cramping. Infections from the IUD can lead to pelvic inflammatory disease, tubal pregnancies, and infertility. The IUD can put us at a higher risk for chlamydia and gonorrhea by causing our vagina to be inflamed and more vulnerable to infection.

Note: Does not protect us from STIs. It can become dislodged, puncturing the uterus or ceasing to be effective birth control. Not recommended for adolescents.

Abstinence: Saying No to Sex

These days, many sex education programs are preaching abstinence—and not always defining what they even mean by this term—with slogans like, "Not everyone's doin' it," and "There's no such thing as safe sex." Their argument is that abstinence is the only way to be safe. Choosing abstinence can be a powerful decision and just right for some of us—but it's incorrect to say that abstinence is our only safe choice, when the above methods are extremely effective. Simply saying "Don't have sex" is not a replacement for being informed about protection and safe sex methods.

Note: Abstinence does not have to mean no sexual pleasure. There are many activities we can substitute for intercourse, for example, kissing, "outercourse" (sexual play without any penetration), and manual stimulation with a partner. *However, abstinence is one hundred percent effective in preventing pregnancy and STIs only when no direct contact with bodily fluids is made.* We can abstain from intercourse and still get an STI from an exchange of bodily fluids during oral sex, anal sex, or contact between genitals. It's also possible to get pregnant with any contact between sperm and our vagina.

Unreliable Methods of Birth Control

Withdrawal

In this method, a guy withdraws his penis from a girl's vagina before ejaculation. Both partners must be in agreement on this method and prepared to deal with an unplanned pregnancy, which can occur in one out of five couples. When no other methods are available, withdrawal is better than nothing. The disadvantage: This method is not very effective because there may be sperm in the pre-ejaculate, which can lead to pregnancy. It also requires a lot of self-control and practice, and it offers no protection from STIs.

Possible side effects: An unwanted pregnancy and/or an STI.

Note: This method is risky business and will leave us feeling very anxious.

Rhythm Method (fertility awareness, periodic abstinence)

Abstaining from sex on our fertile days (when we ovulate or days near ovulation when we can get pregnant) is the only method of birth control outside of abstinence that is approved by the Catholic Church. To do this, we must keep track of our menstrual cycle by checking vaginal discharge and our body temperature. This is not a reliable form of birth control for younger girls because our menstrual cycles are not always regular. This method is more effective in planning a pregnancy than in preventing one. Understanding our cycles is an empowering process but should not be relied upon to prevent pregnancy.

Where to find out about it: There are books available that explain this method and help us figure out our fertility cycles.

Possible side effects: If we are practicing this method, we are putting ourselves at risk for an STI or pregnancy.

Note: If we have irregular menstrual cycles, this method is *extremely* difficult to use.

Pregnancy: Teen Moms

Each year, nearly one million American teens become pregnant.[15] And very few of those pregnant teens will have planned to get pregnant.[16] When we are in a relationship and feel very attached to our partner, the thought of creating a new life together may sound exciting. Taking a reality check at this point can be a smart idea. Imagine life with a baby. How would that be for us? How would it change our lives? How would it change our relationship? Are we ready to be responsible for a helpless human being? Then imagine using birth control every time. That's an easier task than dealing with a pregnancy before we are ready.

- 94 percent of American teens believe that if they became pregnant, they would stay in school; in reality, only 70 percent *eventually* complete high school.
- One-third of pregnant teens in the United States receive inadequate prenatal

care; babies born to young mothers are more likely to have low birth-weights, to have childhood health problems, and to be hospitalized than are those born to older mothers.[17] Bottom line: Unless you want—and are ready for—a baby, *protect yourself.*

Part of me was happy when I found out I was pregnant because I thought it would bring Tom and me closer together.

I met Tom when I was fifteen. He was older, and I didn't know what I was get-ting myself into. He was the first guy I had sex with. We were going to use a condom; he put it on but then took it off. He said, "I know how to do it so you don't get preg-nant." I didn't think I would get pregnant, and I also didn't feel like I could ask him to wear a condom.

Part of me was happy when I found out I was pregnant because I thought it would bring Tom and me closer together. I thought I was in love with him. But when I told him I was pregnant, he said it couldn't be his baby. I was surprised by his reac-tion; we ended up having to go to court and take blood tests to prove he was the father.

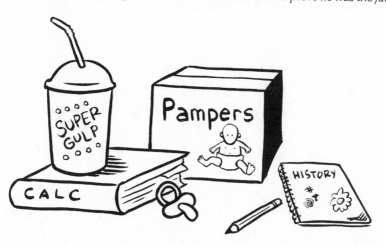

He still doesn't believe it, and he tells people he never had sex with me. I think it's because of his mom and dad; he wants to be a good boy for them. It was a nightmare.

The day I got home from the hospital with my baby, April, I just sat there hold-ing her and looking at her. I thought she was the most amazing and beautiful thing I'd ever seen before. But I didn't think being a mother was going to be so over-whelming and lonely. I didn't go to school during my first year with April, and dur-ing that time I didn't talk to my friends—I didn't have any life. Now that I am back in school, I am tired all the time. April is always in stuff. I have to wait 'til she goes to bed to do my homework because she'll want to sit on my lap or lie on my desk and mess with my papers. By the time she goes to sleep, I'm so tired I usually don't feel like doing my homework. I also hate bringing her to daycare because she always cries when I leave her, and then while I'm at school I think about her.

I haven't dated anyone since first finding out I was pregnant. I'm afraid that a guy might use me like Tom did—just use me for sex. It's been really hard for me to trust guys. Right now I want to finish school and then go on to be a nurse. I want April to grow up feeling loved. Hopefully she's not going to be like me when she's a teenager—I ran wild. I just want her to finish school and go to college.

—Megan, seventeen years old

Reality Check: Teen Pregnancy and Motherhood

Pregnancy is a life-changing experience. Check out these sources on the subject, many in the voices of teenage moms:

Books

Black Teenage Mothers: Pregnancy and Child Rearing from Their Perspective by Constance Willard Williams, Lexington, MA: Lexington Books, 1991.

Dear Diary, I'm Pregnant: Teenagers Talk About Their Pregnancy by Annrenee Englander and Corinne Wilks, Willowdale, ON: Annick Press, 1997.

Going All the Way: Teenage Girls' Tales of Sex, Romance, and Pregnancy by Sharon Thompson, New York: Hill and Wang, 1995.

Nutrition for a Healthy Pregnancy: The Complete Guide to Eating Before, During, and After Your Pregnancy by Elizabeth Somer, New York: Henry Holt, 2002.

Mama Knows Best: African American Wives' Tales, Myths, and Remedies for Mothers and Mothers-To-Be by Chrisena Coleman, New York: Simon & Schuster, 1997.

The Mother Trip: Hip Mama's Guide to Staying Sane in the Chaos of Motherhood by Ariel Gore, Seattle: Seal Press, 2000.

Surviving Teen Pregnancy: Your Choices, Dreams, and Decisions by Shirley Arthur, Buena Park, CA: Morning Glory Press, 1996.

I do believe in birth control, and now we use it.

I was married when I was sixteen, and I had my daughter, Rosa, that same year. I didn't want a baby right away. I didn't use birth control because I didn't think I would get pregnant being so young, but she arrived. I live with my husband, who is twenty-seven. Rosa is two now. I like having a little girl, it's bonita, but at times very difficult because I don't have a lot of experience. Sometimes she is sick, and I don't know what she has. I am still a young girl. Having a baby also affected my friendships because my friends go out and I have to stay in the house with Rosa. The hardest thing is to educate her—I don't know how to talk to her so that she understands

With Child: Wisdom and Traditions for Pregnancy, Birth, and Motherhood by Deborah Jackson, San Francisco: Chronicle Books, 1999.

Films and Videos

Girls Like Us directed by Jane C. Wagner and Tina DiFeliciantonio, 1997.
An ethnically diverse group of four working-class girls strut, flirt, and testify in this vibrant, affecting portrait of teenage girls' experiences of sexuality. Filmed in South Philadelphia and following its subjects from the ages of fourteen to eighteen, *Girls Like Us* reveals the conflicts of growing up female by examining the impact of class, sexism, and violence on the dreams and expectations of young girls.

Girls Town directed by Jim McKay, 1996.
This powerful film is about teenage girls and their relationships with each other and the larger world around them. After a friend commits suicide, the other girls decide to take revenge on the sexist and abusive elements of their community that indirectly led their friend to take her life.

Manny and Lo directed by Lisa Kruger, 1996.
This great movie about the denial involved in a teen pregnancy is also a great sister-bonding flick.

what is right and wrong. I dropped out of school when I had her. I want to finish school so that when she is older I can help her with her school work. I'm starting to take some classes, but it's hard to leave her at daycare because she doesn't want to say good-bye to me and I don't want to separate from her.

I do believe in birth control, and now we use it. But before, when we first got married, I didn't think I would get pregnant. We don't want another baby. I'm glad I have my husband—it's more work for a single mother, and you have to be alone all the time with the baby.

—Carla, eighteen years old

Abortion: The Facts

Each year, women have an estimated 46 million abortions worldwide. Of these, 20 million are clandestine abortions and are generally unsafe. More than three-quarters of all abortions occur in developing countries.[18] Nearly four in ten teen pregnancies (excluding those ending in miscarriages) are terminated by abortion.[19] Abortion is the termination of a pregnancy before the fetus is able to survive outside the uterus. A spontaneous abortion (miscarriage) occurs when natural causes or medical problems end the pregnancy. An induced abortion occurs when the embryo or fetus is intentionally removed through a medical procedure.

Some of us are strongly against induced abortions, a point of view called "pro-life." Some in this group (and some politicians) are trying to limit or reverse a woman's right to an abortion. Others of us, called "pro-choice," believe a woman has the right to decide if she wants to end her pregnancy. Pro-life and pro-choice groups have a long history of debate and conflict. The lack of agreement centers on whether a fetus can be considered a human life. The majority of us feel that abortion is a complicated issue with no easy answer. For example, someone who is pro-choice may believe she would not have an abortion herself but that other women should be able to choose for themselves.

I'm against abortion because I believe it is a life that you are killing.
People don't protect themselves when they should. I know people would get back-alley abortions if abortion wasn't legal, but it is clear to me they are taking a life. Not that they deserve the back-alley abortion, but it should be harder to have abortions because I know people who don't protect themselves. If you use a condom and another method, you won't get pregnant, so I don't see the excuse.

—Sybil, eighteen years old

Everybody I know is pro-choice.

I think I know one or two people who are pro-life. They say, "You are killing a person. You're a murderer." I think a woman should have her own right to decide. It's her body; she should have the choice to do whatever she wants to do with her body. If she's fifteen years old and she's not ready to have a child, why are you going to bring a child into the world? You'll just make the child and the mother suffer. It's not worth it. People will just get abortions anyway. And illegal abortions are really unsafe. Safe abortions need to stay legal.

—Yumi, seventeen years old

What Happens in an Abortion

Often, we talk about whether we are for or against abortion without knowing what it is exactly. There are three ways an induced abortion can be performed—with medicine, by vacuum aspiration (also called dilation and suction curettage, D&C), or through surgery. The following is a list of the basic abortion procedures for different lengths of pregnancy. Before any of these methods, you will need to:

- meet with a counselor at the clinic
- sign a consent form
- give a medical history
- have laboratory tests
- have a physical exam—usually including an ultrasound
- agree to meet with the clinician for a follow-up visit

The first fourteen weeks of pregnancy (first trimester): During the first sixty-three days of the first trimester, we have two options for ending a pregnancy—medical abortion or an abortion by vacuum aspiration. After sixty-three days, vacuum aspiration is the only abortion option during the first trimester.

A medical abortion is a way to end pregnancy without surgery. There are three steps for the medical abortion. In the first step, the clinician gives an injection of methotrexate (which stops the pregnancy in the uterus) or gives a dose of mifepristone in tablet form (this blocks the hormone progesterone, causing the lining of the uterus to break down, ending the pregnancy). In the second step, another medication, called misoprostol in tablet form, is taken, which causes the uterus to contract and empty. The third step is a follow-up visit to the clinician to make sure the abortion is complete, with either an ultrasound or a blood test.

Most women say that it feels like an early miscarriage, with symptoms such as strong cramps, heavy bleeding, abdominal pain, fever and chills, nausea, and diarrhea. The entire process can range from four hours to fourteen days.

An abortion by *vacuum aspiration* is a way to end pregnancy by emptying the uterus with suction. This method is performed in a clinician's office or in a hospital. The contents of the uterus (embryo or fetus, placenta, and uterine lining) are vacuumed out with a soft plastic tube. Before insertion, a medication or special dilator may be inserted to help open the cervix. After seven weeks, a larger tube is used and may involve more discomfort or cramping. A spoonlike instrument, called a curette, may also be used to scrape the uterus lining to make sure there is no tissue left.

The entire procedure takes around fifteen minutes, and then you rest in a recovery room for about an hour. There may be bleeding off and on for a couple weeks afterward. Some women have cramps and pass a few large blood clots for up to ten days after the procedure. Most women say they feel pain similar to strong menstrual cramps, and for others it is more uncomfortable. A local anesthetic is usually used.

Thirteen to sixteen weeks (early second trimester): At this stage in the pregnancy, a larger suction tube and curette are used to remove the contents of the uterus. In some abortions, laminaria sticks or osmotic devices (resembling small tampons) are used to dilate (stretch) the cervix over several hours or a few days in order to allow the passage of the suction tube. These devices are usually placed inside the vagina the day before the scheduled appointment and worn overnight.

Sixteen to twenty-four weeks (later second trimester): The procedures used at this stage are similar to those used in an early second-trimester abortion, except that the instruments are larger and the abortion takes longer. In unusual circumstances, labor and delivery of the fetus is caused by a special fluid injected through the abdomen into the amniotic sac surrounding the fetus. Or the abdomen and uterus are cut open and the contents of the uterus removed.

Teens have a high rate of late abortions (around the twentieth week), which carry more risks than abortions during the earlier weeks of pregnancy.[20] Reasons we may put off getting an abortion include denial, being afraid to tell anyone, financial obstacles, and difficulty in deciding whether or not to abort. *The earlier we get an abortion, the safer, less painful, and less expensive it is.*

If we are deciding whether or not to have an abortion, it is helpful to discuss the issue with an adult we trust and are comfortable with, such as a parent, friend, or counselor from school, church, or another community organization. Clinics, such as Planned Parenthood or our local women's health center, can also help us in our decision. They do not tell us what to do, but will talk to us about all the choices we have, like abortion, adoption, or keeping the baby. They will also explain what happens during an abortion and answer any questions we may have. After having an abortion, we may also find it helpful to discuss our feelings and thoughts with a counselor, parent, or trusted friend as we move on from the experience.

Myth: Eating certain foods, exercising vigorously, or using other do-it-yourself techniques can lead to abortion.

Reality: These methods are dangerous. A home remedy can make us ill or have side effects that we are not prepared for. And inserting objects (e.g., a wire coat hanger or knitting needle) into the uterus to induce an abortion can lead to death from infection or bleeding.

Abortion Clinics Online is a directory service that provides a complete list of abortion providers in every state. Find them online at www.gynpages.com. Or call Planned Parenthood at (800) 230-PLAN to reach the Planned Parenthood clinic nearest you.

I didn't have sex for two years after my abortion because the experience was so emotional.

When I was sixteen, I started vomiting every day and didn't know what was the matter. My mom asked if I was possibly pregnant, and I said "no," but I knew I could be. My boyfriend had lied to me and said I couldn't get pregnant if he pulled out before coming, and I wanted to believe him. My dad took me to the hospital to get tests to see what was wrong with me. I was pregnant. I told the doctor I wanted to have an abortion. I didn't tell my father; he thought it was the flu. When I got home, I told my mother. She supported my decision to get an abortion. I told my boyfriend I was pregnant and that I was going to get an abortion. He went along with my decision. We stopped dating each other soon after that.

I got the abortion at Planned Parenthood one week after finding out I was pregnant. I went with my mom, and we met with a counselor. The counselor explained the procedure and the other options, like keeping the baby or giving it up for adoption. Then she asked my mom to leave the room. She was really nice. She asked if I was sure this was what I wanted to do and said she would support me with whatever decision I wanted to make. I was sure I wanted to have the abortion, so we went ahead with it. First they gave me a shot in the cervix, which hurt a lot. Then they put a tube in my vagina that sucked the fetus out. That part didn't hurt.

Afterward, I slept. When I woke up, I felt much better, not nauseous, and relieved about the decision.

I knew I had done the right thing. I was too young. I couldn't have handled having a baby at that age. My parents would have supported me, but the baby would have been my responsibility. I didn't want my parents to pay for me and my baby. I

History of Abortion

Abortion has been practiced throughout history, and the disagreement over whether or not it should be practiced is nothing new. In ancient Greece (around 300 BC), people believed the fetus had no soul, and Aristotle and others recommended abortion as a way to limit family size. In contrast, in ancient Assyria, the practice led to harsh penalties.[1]

In the United States, before the mid-1800s, abortion was not a crime under common law. Advertisements for abortion services appeared in respectable newspapers, journals, and magazines. State laws prohibiting abortion began to be passed in the 1820s, when first Connecticut and then twenty other states banned abortions after twenty weeks of pregnancy— when women were said to be able to feel the fetus move.[2] In 1869, Pope Pius IX issued a decree declaring abortion sinful and banned it entirely. By 1900, abortions were illegal all over America. For the next seventy years, women had to resort to dangerous illegal abortions if they wanted to end a pregnancy. Some women could afford to leave the country for an abortion or pay a doctor under the table. But many women suffered hemorrhage, infection, and even death from botched illegal abortions.

In the 1960s, a few states liberalized their abortion laws, and in 1970, four states legalized abortion: Alaska, Hawaii, New York, and Washington. In January 1973, the Supreme Court ruled in the case of Roe v. Wade that women have the legal right to choose whether or not to have an abortion. This ruling removed all legal restrictions on abortion during the first three months of pregnancy and gave the states the right to regulate abortions during the third to sixth months of pregnancy, but only to protect the woman's health. In the 1992 Casey decision, the Supreme Court ruled that individual states could pass laws concerning abortions in their states, though abortion itself remained legal. Restrictions okayed by the court include a twenty-four hour *also have dreams, like going to college, and I don't think I could have done that with a baby. Now I'm nineteen, and there is no way I can imagine having a three-year-old—that would be so tough. I don't ever doubt my decision to have an abortion.*

I couldn't talk about my abortion with anyone for a long time. After the initial shock wore off, I felt more comfortable with the experience. I was then able to talk

waiting period between counseling and abortion, counseling to advise not getting an abortion, and parental consent or notification laws (see below).

Currently, members of Congress are seeking to pass something called the "Child Custody Protection Act." The bill would make it a federal crime to transport a minor across state lines for an abortion unless the parental involvement requirements of her home state had been met. If the bill were enacted, persons convicted would be subject to imprisonment, fines, and civil suits.

Parental Consent/Notification Laws

Thirty-four states have parental involvement laws in effect for girls under eighteen years of age. Some of these laws require a parent, and sometimes both parents, to sign a consent form in order for the girl to have an abortion. Other laws require that the parents be notified when their daughter seeks an abortion. If we do not want to talk to our parents about having an abortion, parental consent laws may make us postpone getting an abortion or force us to choose an unsafe, illegal abortion. However, despite this objection, an ABC News/*Washington Post* poll found that 79 percent of Americans were in favor of parental consent laws—a far greater number than those who oppose abortion in general.[3]

Judicial Bypass

If we live in a state that has parental consent laws, we can still get a legal abortion without our parents' consent. A judge can give us permission to have an abortion if we prove to the judge that we are mature enough to make the decision ourselves, or if we explain why we cannot get consent from our parents. If we have no other option, going through a judicial bypass procedure is worth it to avoid the risks of an illegal abortion. It can be intimidating, so we should bring a close friend for support.

about it, which helped. I didn't have sex for two years after that because the experience was so emotional. It was hard for me to trust a guy, and I was afraid of getting pregnant.

—Kelly, nineteen years old

after her abortion

she lay on her bed
in the hotel,
staring
at the painting of shells.
he kissed her,
brought her a plate
of scrambled eggs.
then the names rose
from her tired womb:
names for the little worm
she had killed
flying around her
in circles, like tiny
buzzards, cruel winged children,
chanting until she puked.
in the bathroom that night
she drew the shower curtain closed
with such sadness that he started to cry.
she sat on the toilet watching him sob,
watching him wonder
whether or not to touch her,
to turn his back, to grieve.

—Robin, seventeen years old

I thought about the baby, and a part of me missed it.

I got pregnant this year with the guy I was dating because the condom ripped—it had been in his wallet for a long time. I broke up with him after I found out I was pregnant. I didn't tell him about the pregnancy until after the abortion because I was scared. I'm the type of person who keeps things to myself. I didn't talk about my abortion with anyone. My parents still don't know to this day.

I knew I was going to have an abortion. I didn't have the resources to raise a child on my own—mentally or money-wise. I went to a health clinic, and a counselor there told me about other options, but I was set on having an abortion. The abortion was painful to go through. It hurt because I cramped a lot and bled for a while afterwards. After it was over, I was relieved but also sad. I thought about the baby, and a part of me missed it. It's a child I helped make.

I told my ex-boyfriend afterwards, and he cried and said he wished he could have been there with me. He was sorry and felt bad. We are still close friends. I didn't have sex for a year and a half after. I needed to get over the mental part of the abortion. The fact that the condom broke made me think, "This is not happening again." I can't have a one-night fling or have sex if I'm not sure. I have to know that I like the guy I'm going to have sex with. To me, sex is tied to emotions and how I feel toward the person, which brings about sexual attraction. If I can't feel close to the person I'm fooling around with, it's not going to bring enjoyment to me, so why bother? The next time I had sex, I was ready and sure about it. If I ever get pregnant again, I would talk to someone about it and tell the father. It made it a lot harder for me, keeping everything to myself. When things are tough, I form a shell around myself and don't tell people what's going on. I don't want to keep doing that—I want to be able to get support from others.

—Estelle, eighteen years old

Emergency Contraception

Emergency Contraception is not a substitute for birth control, but is an option in an emergency situation (for example, if our birth control method fails or if we have been sexually assaulted).

There are two types of emergency contraception available:

The Emergency Contraceptive Pill (ECP) method: The ECP, or "morning after pill," uses a high dose of combined oral contraceptives (OCs) to prevent conception. The OC method is effective if used within seventy-two hours after unprotected intercourse. (Used within five days of intercourse, it has a 75 percent effectiveness rate.) ECP is available from your doctor, hospital, or birth-control clinic by prescription. The side effects can be strong: nausea, breast tenderness, and alterations in the menstrual cycle. Other more serious but uncommon side effects include blood clots, heart attack, migraine headaches, and high blood pressure.

The Intrauterine Device (IUD) method: This method involves the insertion of an IUD into the uterus by a clinician. The IUD creates an unfriendly environment for egg and sperm. The IUD must be inserted within seven days of unprotected sex. Side effects of IUD insertion may include abdominal discomfort, vaginal bleeding, or spotting and infection. Possible side effects of IUD use include heavy menstrual flow, cramping, infection, infertility, and uterine puncture.

> For more information call the Emergency Contraception Hotline, (800) 584-9911.

Sexually Transmitted Infections

Sexually transmitted infections (STIs) affect both males and females and are transmitted through intimate contact with someone who already has an infection, especially during unprotected oral, anal, and vaginal sex. The bacteria or virus that causes an STI almost always enters the body through a mucous membrane—the warm, moist surfaces of the vagina, anus, and mouth. If we have one STI, it does not mean we can't get another. And being cured of an STI does not mean we can't catch it again. But STIs are not an inevitable part of sex: If we and our partner consistently use condoms and/or dental dams, are exclusive partners (monogamous), and get regular checkups with the doctor, then we can usually be healthy and STI-free.

Myth: Boys are more at risk for STIs than girls are.

Reality: It is easier for a male to pass an STI, including the HIV virus that causes AIDS (see the next section on AIDS), to a female than it is for a female to pass it to a male. If we think about the mechanics involved, it makes sense: During vaginal intercourse, the male puts his penis inside a female's vagina, ejaculates, and then withdraws. Any bacteria or virus is much more likely to remain with the female than with the male. In a single act of unprotected sex with an infected partner, a female is twice as likely as a male to get gonorrhea, chlamydia, or hepatitis B.[21]

Myth: It is rare for a young person to get an STI.

Reality: STIs are very common among teenagers. Not only do two-thirds of all STIs occur in people twenty-five years of age or younger, but one in four new STI infections occurs in teenagers.[22]

STIs cause discomfort, may be life-threatening, and can lead to infertility. Of the more than twenty-five types that have been identified, most are caused by bacteria (for example, gonorrhea, syphilis, and chlamydia) and are curable with antibiotics.

Other STIs are caused by viruses (for example, genital herpes, human papillomavirus virus or HPV, hepatitis B, and AIDS) and are not curable, but the symptoms may be alleviated with the proper medical care. A few STIs are caused by protozoa (trichomoniasis) and other tiny insects (for example, crabs, scabies, and pubic lice). These STIs are curable with antibiotics or topical creams and lotions. Whether or not we are sexually active, we should know about STIs because knowledge is power.

Common STIs

It is very common to be infected with an STI long before we can see any symptoms. Annual pelvic exams are the best way to find out if we have an STI and to receive early treatment.

Three STIs (human papillomavirus, trichomoniasis, and chlamydia) accounted for 88 percent of all new cases of STIs among fifteen- to twenty-four-year-olds in the year 2000.[23] Arm yourself with information on these and some other common STIs:

- **Chlamydia:** This is the most common STI. First symptoms usually appear two weeks to one month after being infected: pain during urination, vaginal itching or increased vaginal discharge, abdominal pain, bleeding between periods, and low-grade fever. Four-fifths of infected women do not show any symptoms. At its worst, chlamydia can lead to infertility, blindness, and pneumonia. It can be cured with antibiotics.

- **Genital herpes (herpes):** First symptoms usually appear within two weeks of being infected: a cluster of tender, painful blisters in the genital area, painful urination, and often swollen glands and fever. Infection may be linked to cervical cancer. The presence of sores may increase vulnerability to other STIs, including HIV, and can damage babies during birth. Another strain of herpes infects the mouth area. However, both of these strains can be passed from the mouth to the genitals and vice versa. No cure is available, though there are medications to alleviate the painful symptoms; outbreaks usually recur.

- **Gonorrhea (dose, clap, drip):** First symptoms usually appear two to ten days after being infected: white or yellow discharge, painful urination, and lower abdominal pain, especially after your period. But an infected woman may show no symptoms. Gonorrhea can eventually lead to infertility or blindness if the eyes become infected. It can be cured with antibiotics.

- **Hepatitis-B (serum hepatitis):** People who are infected are often asymptomatic (no symptoms appear). If symptoms do appear, they include low-grade fever, fatigue, general aches, loss of appetite, nausea and vomiting, abdominal pain, and a yellowish hue to the skin and eyes. Hepatitis-B is a serious STI that can be caught even from saliva exchange through kissing. It is transmitted through bodily secretions (tears, sweat, saliva, vaginal secretions, and semen), contaminated blood, and shared needles. Hepatitis-B can lead to liver disease. No cure is available, but there is a vaccine to prevent infections.

※ **Human Papillomavirus (HPV, genital warts):** One to three months after contact, this virus may cause warts on the genitals, anus, or throat. People who are infected often show no symptoms, but infected cells can be detected through a Pap smear. Infection can lead to increased risk for cervical and vaginal cancer. A health care provider can remove warts as well as infected cells; regular follow-up exams and Pap smears are necessary to check if the virus is dormant.

※ **Syphilis (syph, pox, bad blood):** First symptoms usually appear three weeks after infection: In the first stage, a painless blister or sore appears on the genitals, anus, or lips; the second stage includes a rash or mucous patches, some hair loss, a sore throat, and swollen glands. Stage-two symptoms may recur for up to two years. If left untreated, third-stage syphilis can lead to brain damage, insanity, paralysis, heart disease, and death. Syphilis can also harm unborn babies. It can be cured with antibiotics.

※ **Trichomoniasis (trick, TV):** First symptoms appear one to four weeks after infection: frothy discharge from the vagina, very itchy, burning, and red genitals, and pain during sexual intercourse. Infected males usually show no symptoms. It can be cured with antibiotics.

※ **Pelvic Inflammatory Disease (PID):** This is an infection of the upper genital tract (the pelvis area, between the hip bones) that occurs once we have an STI. Disease-causing organisms migrate upward from the urethra and cervix into the upper genital tract. Many different organisms can cause PID, but most cases are associated with gonorrhea and genital chlamydial infections. Bacteria normally present in small numbers in the vagina and cervix also may play a role. If left untreated, it can cause infertility or more frequent periods. Severe cases may even spread to the liver and kidneys, causing dangerous internal bleeding, lung failure, and death. Each year in the United States, more than one million women experience an episode of acute PID, with the rate of infection highest among teenagers.[24]

HIV/AIDS

The HIV/AIDS pandemic is one of the most important and urgent
public health challenges facing governments and civil societies
around the world. Adolescents are at the centre of the pandemic
in terms of transmission, impact, and potential for changing the
attitudes and behaviors that underlie this disease.

—World Health Organization

AIDS (acquired immune deficiency syndrome) is caused by the human immunodeficiency virus (HIV). HIV is passed from one person to another by virus-contaminated
bodily fluids—semen, vaginal secretions, breast milk, or blood. The virus typically
gains entrance to the bloodstream through sexual contact or intravenous (IV) drug
use with a contaminated needle. HIV can also be passed from mother to child during pregnancy, delivery, and breastfeeding. When someone is infected with HIV, it
may be six months or longer before a test will show that they are infected (HIV positive), and years before they show any physical signs of AIDS. The virus causes a
breakdown of the immune system, which ordinarily protects us against infections.
Because of the collapse of these immune defenses, people with HIV typically come
down with a variety of deadly infections. Although new treatments have evolved in
recent years, there is still no cure or effective vaccine for HIV.

Current statistics on HIV/AIDS indicate that one-half of all new HIV infections
worldwide occur among young people ages fifteen to twenty-four.[25] Advocates for
Youth states that: "Every minute, five young people worldwide become infected with
HIV/AIDS. This is over 7,000 young people each day."[26] The vast majority of young
people who are HIV positive do not know that they are infected, and few who are
engaging in sex know the HIV status of their partners."[27]

Given these facts, it is extremely important that we understand our own risk for
HIV and AIDS and arm ourselves with the latest information. As adolescents and as
human beings, when it comes to our sexual health, we have the right to information,
a range of services, and a safe and supportive environment. HIV/AIDS flourishes
where human rights are not protected, particularly in countries or areas where adolescents do not go to school and do not have access to information about AIDS or to
opportunities to develop the life skills that they need to turn this information into
action. Frequently, they also do not have access to services that take their specific
needs into consideration.[28]

What can we do?

- Protect ourselves first. We cannot help someone else if we do not take care of ourselves first. This means making healthy choices by understanding how HIV/AIDS is transmitted and how we can best protect ourselves.
- Know the facts on HIV/AIDS. Great places for online information about HIV/AIDS include: www.thebody.com, www.cdc.gov/hiv, and www.aidsmap.com.
- Do something to help. HIV/AIDS is a worldwide problem, and we can make a difference. We may want to volunteer or find work doing activities such as education, outreach, and advocacy. Or we may simply want to share what we know with others in our lives.
- Pick up the phone. For specific questions or concerns about AIDS, call the Centers for Disease Control's free national HIV/AIDS hotline at (800) 342-2437. If you speak Spanish, call (800) 344-7432. If you are deaf, call (800) 243-7889.

Myth: It's mostly gay people who get HIV.

Reality: Most new HIV cases today are among heterosexuals. Statistically, lesbians are less likely to contract HIV (but there are safer-sex measures lesbians can and should take). If we have sex with both males and females, the chances of contracting HIV are the same as for heterosexuals.

Myth: If you're not sexually active, you can't get HIV.

Reality: We can get HIV from any exchange of infected blood, semen, or vaginal secretions. This means that you can be infected through non-sexual contact, such as the sharing of an HIV-contaminated needle.

Myth: You can get HIV from everyday contact like hugging and kissing, from public drinking fountains, or from mosquito bites.

Reality: To date, there are no recorded cases of HIV infection from these contacts. There are only three known ways for getting HIV: 1) unprotected anal, oral, or vaginal sex with an infected partner; 2) contaminated blood transfusions or IV drug use; 3) birth and breastfeeding by an infected mother.

Ways to Reduce Our Risk of Getting an STI

There are several steps we can take to protect ourselves from sexually transmitted infections. If we've chosen to be sexually active, we need to know how to take care of ourselves and then follow through on that knowledge.

- Use condoms (put it on before sex, do not remove until the end, and hold it to the penis as he pulls out of your vagina).
- Talk to your partner about his or her past sexual practices and whether he or she has any STIs. You may both want to be tested and then make a mutual decision to be monogamous. The fewer partners you both have, the lower your chances are of getting an STI.
- Ask about any discharges, sores, or rashes you see on your partner.
- Wash your genitals with soap and water before and after sexual intercourse, and have your partner wash too. Also, urinate after intercourse.
- Avoid "ping pong" infection, when you and your partner give the same STI back and forth to each other. If one partner has an STI, the other partner must be treated at the same time to avoid re-infection.
- Get regular pelvic exams.
- If you are concerned or think you have symptoms, ask to be tested for STIs.

I don't think sex has to be scary if you use a condom.

These days, sex is always equated with fear, death and AIDS. There's always a consequence to it. It hasn't been like that for me. I think that telling you the consequences of sex doesn't make people not want to have sex—you know we all have hormones. Curriculums that say that abstinence is the only effective method to avoid pregnancy and disease make people more afraid to talk to their partner about sex and using condoms.

—Alex, fifteen years old

What Should We Do If We Think We Have an STI?

Only about half of us with STIs notice any signs of an infection. We can be infected but not have any symptoms for a long time or not recognize the signs when we do have them. Getting tested for STIs can tell us if we have an STI long before we notice the physical symptoms.

If we think we have been exposed to an STI, experience possible symptoms, or have concerns, the most important thing for us to do is discuss this with a health care provider and get tested. Diagnosis of sexually transmitted infections requires laboratory tests and/or physical examination. We cannot assume that we will be tested during a routine pelvic exam or in a general visit to the doctor, as many providers do not automatically test for STIs; nor will they test for every STI, unless they notice—or we mention—something suspicious. This is of concern since some STIs have no symptoms. Therefore, it is important for us to speak up for ourselves and our health. In speaking with our doctor, we may say something like: "I'm worried that I may have one or several STIs. I had unprotected intercourse (or anal or oral sex) during the last three months." If we are not comfortable with our regular doctor or gynecologist, we can go to a health clinic, like Planned Parenthood or our local women's health clinic. And, we should remember that some awkwardness is better than simply hoping our concerns are wrong or waiting for symptoms to go away, and ending up with a serious disease and long-term consequences.

Several STIs can be cured, usually with antibiotics, and others can be controlled. If we think we or our sexual partners are infected, we should either have sex using a barrier method (the male condom is the most effective contraception for preventing the spread of STIs) or abstain from sex until we have been tested or are sure that we are cured. If we do have an STI, it is best to inform all past and present sexual partners who may have been exposed to infection.

Conditions That Are Not STIs

The following conditions are not STIs but are sometimes confused with them:

❋ **Vaginitis:** Overgrowth of normal microorganisms in the vagina that causes itching, burning, and swelling. The most common types are: yeast infections, which are caused by a yeast fungus called candida and produce a discharge that looks like cottage cheese and smells sweet or breadlike; and bacterial vaginosis, which is caused by bacteria and produces a gray, fishy-smelling discharge. Causes of vaginitis include: stress, lack of sleep, inadequate diet, infrequent bathing or washing of the vaginal area, antibiotic use, birth control pills, douching, and sexual intercourse with a partner who is infected with an STI. Yeast infections are usually treated with an antimicrobial cream or pill (some creams can be purchased at the drugstore without a prescription).

❋ **Urinary tract infection:** A bacterial infection in the urethra (the tube from the bladder to the outside of body) that causes painful urination. Urinary tract infections can be caused by lack of bathing or washing of the genitals, sexual intercourse, and withholding urination. It is a good idea to pee before and after intercourse to decrease your chances of infection. Urinary tract infections are usually treated with antibiotics.

There are situations when we cannot protect ourselves from STIs. If we are forced to have sex with someone and that person does not use a condom, it is very important that we seek medical help right away and get examined for any possible infections.

For specific questions and referrals to clinics, call the Centers for Disease Control's free national STI hotline at (800) 227-8922.

Sexual Assault

Sometimes we may not have control over a sexual situation. Whenever we are forced by another person to participate in sexual behavior, this is considered sexual assault. When we are in a relationship that has a pattern of intimidation and abuse, this is considered a violent or abusive relationship. We are all affected, directly or indirectly, by violence, rape, and abuse. At least one woman in three around the world has been beaten, coerced into sex, or abused during her lifetime. The abuser is most often someone she knows or a member of her own family.[29] Whether or not we have been assaulted or abused or know someone who has been, the fear of rape has an impact on our lives. We are told not to walk alone at night, to be suspicious of strangers—especially men—and to be cautious on first dates. We share stories of childhoods traumatized by abuse at the hands of our caretakers and wonder how the cycle can be broken.

Women are doing things to combat physical and psychological violence against women and the fear and limits it creates. "Take Back the Night" marches are held yearly in cities around the country as women march together at night through areas that might be dangerous if walked through alone. Rallies are held to allow people to speak about their experiences of sexual assault and rape, and to voice both their rage over having to live in fear and their strength in moving on. These marches and rallies help to empower and inform us. Dismantling the myths around rape and sharing our stories help us put rape in its place—as an event that is not our fault, and as something that is totally unacceptable.

Myth: A woman who gets raped must have "asked for it." She must have led the guy on with her skimpy clothing, walked alone late at night, or sent out mixed signals with her flirtations.

Reality: Women do not ask to be raped. Even if we walk naked into a bar, no one has the right to have sex with us when we say no.

Myth: Rapes mostly happen late at night, in dark alleys, and are committed by strangers.

Reality: The majority of rapes occur in the context of dating: A survey of adolescent and college students revealed that date rape accounted for 67 percent of sexual assaults.[30]

In addition to empowering ourselves and others with support and information, it can be helpful to plan ahead. The following is a list of ideas to keep our dates safe:[31]

- Consider double-dating the first few times you go out with a new person.
- Before leaving on a date, know the exact plans for the evening and make sure a parent or friend knows these plans and what time to expect you home. Let your date know that you are expected to call or tell that person when you get in.
- Be aware of your decreased ability to react under the influence of alcohol or drugs.
- If you leave a party with someone you do not know well, make sure you tell another person that you are leaving and with whom. Ask a friend to call and make sure you arrived home safely.
- Assert yourself when necessary. Be firm and straightforward in your relationships.
- Trust your instincts. If a situation makes you uncomfortable, try to be calm and think of a way to remove yourself from the situation.

The following resources are available for support: National Domestic Violence Hotline at (800) 799-7233; the twenty-four-hour confidential rape hotline sponsored by Rape, Abuse & Incest National Network at (800) 656-HOPE; and the National Victim Center at (800) FYI-CALL, in operation from 8:30 AM to 5:30 PM EST. These hotlines can also help us find assistance and resources in our local communities.

For those of us who have not been assaulted, we wonder what would happen to our lives if we were. The courage of those of us who have been raped or assaulted and now speak out about it shows us that life does continue and we can heal.

Definitions of Sexual Assault

※ *Rape* is nonconsensual (not agreed upon) oral, anal, or vaginal penetration obtained by force, by threat of bodily harm, or when the victim is unable to give consent—for example, when the victim has passed out from drug or alcohol use.

※ *Sexual assault* includes rape and other forced unwanted sexual interaction, such as touching and kissing.

※ *Date rape* or *acquaintance rape* is when the victim knows and has interacted with the rapist before the attack. The majority of rapes are committed by someone the victim knows.[1]

※ *Incest* is sexual contact that occurs between family members. Often this contact is not consensual and involves an older male with a younger female relative. Sexual contact may include a variety of verbal and/or physical behaviors; penetration is not necessary for the experience to count as incest.

※ *Sexual abuse* is sexual contact (with or without force) with an individual, usually committed by someone in a position of authority over that individual, such as a relative, family friend, doctor, teacher, coach, or babysitter.

※ *Sexual harassment* is any unwanted sexual attention, such as touching, patting, sexual comments, or pressure to go out on a date. The harasser may have power over the victim, such as a boss harassing an employee or a professor harassing a student.

Definition of Dating Violence

In dating violence, one partner tries to maintain power and control over the other through abuse, including:

※ any kind of physical violence or threat of physical violence to get control

※ emotional or mental abuse, such as playing mind games, making you feel crazy, or constantly putting you down and criticizing you

※ sexual abuse, including making you do anything you don't want to, refusing to have safer sex, or making you feel bad about yourself sexually

It wasn't until I talked to a counselor about it that I understood it wasn't my fault.

This guy, George, almost raped me. He did things to me despite the fact that I told him no. It was the worst experience of my life.

It was my fifteenth birthday, and I was in a fight with my best friend, Lynn. I was hanging out with George because I thought he was my friend. He totally took advantage of the situation. He brought beer with him and kept telling me to "drink up." And then he took me to a separate room to watch TV. George locked the door and started touching me. I struggled and said, "No, I don't want to do this. I don't think this should happen." He kept grabbing me and said, "Oh, it's okay, don't worry about it. We'll just do it anyway." He ripped off all my clothes, held my knees down, and I couldn't do anything. He was a big football player. I didn't know what was going on. My mind was racing: "Didn't I say no?" Then all of a sudden: Bang, bang, bang, bang on the door, right after he said he was going to have sex with me. He got up, threw my clothes in my face, put on his clothes, and unlocked the door.

My friend Lynn came in, and I was in tears. I had put on my clothes, but I was crying really hard. I told her what happened, and she thought I was lying. She couldn't deal with it. She said, "I know George, and I know he wouldn't do anything like that." Later, I started to wonder myself, "Well, maybe it didn't really happen like that. Maybe something was different, yeah, yeah, maybe this happened . . . " I didn't tell anyone else because I didn't want them to tell me I was a liar.

The whole experience affected me for a long time. I used to come home and cry hysterically and punch myself in the stomach. I was so out of it emotionally. I was not stable, and I was so ashamed. I would cry in my bathroom—sitting on the floor.

At the time, I was unable to understand that it wasn't my fault. It wasn't until the next summer that I talked to a counselor about it and had new insights. She told me I was not to blame. That summer, I didn't want to date anyone or let a guy touch me. I just wanted to concentrate on becoming a healthy human being. Even though what happened was the worst experience of my life, I learned so much about myself because of it. Horrible things happen to you, but you become a stronger person for it.

—Dalia, sixteen years old

I feel like I'm getting stronger. I'm going to have a successful future.

From when I was five to ten years old, I was sexually molested by the boy next door. His name was Danny, and he was five years older than me. He was someone I grew up with; he was like a brother to me. The first time it happened, we were playing hide and seek. He shut the door and locked it behind me. Danny told me that we were "switching peepees." He would put his "peepee" in my "peepee." It hurt me down there. I didn't feel comfortable with how he grabbed me, kissed me, and did *all this stuff I didn't understand. I didn't feel good inside—someone was touching my body like nobody else did.*

I tried to tell my mom, "Mommy, Danny and me were switching peepees." But she didn't pay any attention to it. She said, "You don't know what you are talking about." As I got older, it bothered me more and more. I would tell Danny to stop, but he wouldn't listen. When I was ten, I found the strength to tell him, "It's over, you can't do this anymore." He said, "Come on, come on," but I said, "No." After this, I was able to stand my ground, and he finally left me alone.

My experience with Danny made me feel like I couldn't trust anyone. In seventh grade, I couldn't relate to the other students. Some people thought I was slow because I was always nervous. I had a lot of fear of rejection and bad self-esteem. I hated my body. When I look at pictures now, there was nothing wrong with my body, but back then I didn't see it that way.

Then, in high school, I had a boyfriend who taught me, "Guys should respect you. Guys should be proud of holding your hand. You don't deserve anything bad." It woke me up. After that, I never let a guy take advantage of me the way Danny did.

I didn't start telling people until this year. I've been doing a lot of art work, and I find it helps me to think about myself. I started meeting with a counselor, and I've been writing in a journal. All of this freed me up to talk about my experience. Now that I'm telling my friends, I find that some of them have similar experiences. I feel like I'm getting stronger. I'm going to have a successful future.

—Tanya, eighteen years old

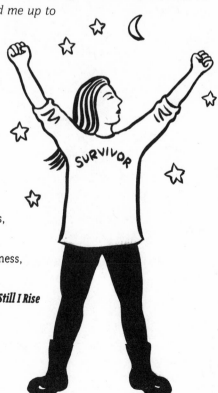

You may shoot me with your words,
You may cut me with your eyes,
You may kill me with your hatefulness,
But still, like air, I'll rise.

—Maya Angelou, "Still I Rise," *And Still I Rise*

Recovering from Sexual Assault

Sexual assault can be a traumatic experience, but it is possible to reclaim our lives. The path to healing is different for everyone. The following books and organizations can offer hope and guidance along the way:

Books

The Courage to Heal: A Guide for Women Survivors of Child Sexual Abuse by Ellen Bass and Laura Davis, New York: HarperPerennial Library, 1994.

Daybreak: Meditations for Women Survivors of Sexual Abuse by Maureen Brady, New York: HarperCollins, 1991.

Defending Ourselves: A Guide to Prevention, Self-Defense, and Recovery from Rape by Rosalind Wiseman, New York: Noonday Press, 1994.

The Gift of Fear: Survival Signs That Protect Us from Violence by Gavin De Becker, New York: Dell, 1998.

I Never Called It Rape by Robin Warshaw, New York: Harper and Row, 1998.

I Will Survive: The African American Guide to Healing From Sexual Assault and Abuse by Lori Robinson, Emeryville, CA: Seal Press, 2002.

In Love and In Danger: A Teen's Guide to Breaking Free of Abusive Relationships by Barrie Levy, Seattle: Seal Press, 1997.

Intimate Betrayal: Understanding and Responding to the Trauma of Acquaintance Rape by Vernon R. Wiehe and Ann L. Richards, Thousand Oaks, CA: Sage Publications, 1995.

Invisible Girls: The Truth About Sexual Abuse by Dr. Patti Feuereisen and Caroline Pincus, Emeryville, CA: Seal Press, 2005.

Journey to Wholeness: Healing from the Trauma of Rape by Vicki Aranow et al., Holmes Beach, FL: Learning Publications, 2000.

She Who Was Lost Is Remembered: Healing from Incest Through Creativity edited by Louise M. Wisechild, Seattle: Seal Press, 1991.

Voices of Rape edited by Janet Bode, New York: Franklin Watts, 1998.

When Something Feels Wrong: A Survival Guide About Abuse for Young People by Deanna S. Pledge, Minneapolis, MN: Free Spirit Publishing, 2003.

Organizations

Anti-Violence Resource Guide

Created by V-Day and feminist.com, this resource provides a detailed list of organizations and resources for ending violence against women.
website: www.feminist.com/antiviolence

National Coalition Against Sexual Assault

PO Box 21378
Washington, D.C. 20009
phone: (202) 483-7165

Rape Crisis Centers

Rape crisis centers exist in many cities and many offer a hotline that anyone can call in order to talk to a trained counselor about experiences with rape, assault, or abuse. Volunteers are available to accompany and advocate for survivors dealing with the aftermath of an assault. Check your phone book for the rape crisis center nearest you.

Self-Defense Classes

Call your local YWCA or any local women's center to find a self-defense class. You can also try to find a class through your school, a local college, a martial arts studio, or an adult education program. There are also books available on how to defend yourself (see list above for some ideas). Read them with friends so you can try out some maneuvers.

Survivors of Incest Anonymous

SIA is a free twelve-step self-help peer program for incest survivors. SIA will mail you extensive literature (free if you can't afford it) and its bimonthly newsletter. To locate programs in your area, request a directory of meetings from the national SIA number below or look at its website.
PO Box 21817
Baltimore, MD 21222
phone: (410) 433-2365
website: www.siawso.org

Taking Charge

Being in charge of our sexuality means being informed about safer sexual practices and making thoughtful choices. It is important to think about our sexual rights and limits before we are in the heat of the moment. Make plans ahead of time: "I'm not going to have sex with this person until I'm ready," "We are going to use a condom no matter what happens," or "I'm going to ask about her sexual past before we fool around." Deciding on our boundaries and what's important to us ahead of time leaves us empowered and feeling in control of the moment. We can share our concerns about sex with friends and support them in their choices. We should remember that sexual assault is never our fault and know that we can take charge of our own healing and support others in theirs. There is strength in numbers and in being vocal.

Getting information about the contraception choices available to us, about common STIs, about our reproductive rights, and about the reality of pregnancy is important to all of us, no matter what stage of sexual exploration we are in. Don't buy into myths—get informed and feel powerful.

7

Feminism
What Is It, and Do We Care?

To me, "feminism" isn't defined by Gloria Steinem or anyone else.
It's something I think I create for myself—and it's the whole ideology with which I look at things.

—Nicole, fifteen years old

I don't want to be treated differently from boys.
There's no one thing women "should" be; they should just be allowed to be who they are. I hate when boys look at you and instead of seeing a person or a mind, they see a dumb victim or they try to sweet-talk you. I'm blunt with them, and I'll tell them, "I'll pound you if you treat me like that."

—Zoe, seventeen years old

Feminism in America has come a long way since the 1800s, when the primary focus was on women gaining the right to vote. Now that we can vote and stand on more equal ground, some assume that women have "arrived" and the need for a feminist movement is over. But is the need for an active women's movement dead and buried? Consider the following:

- When you turn on the news, you aren't likely to see a gray-haired anchorwoman delivering the news (97 percent of TV anchors over the age of forty are men!).[1] Also, if you see wrinkles on a newscaster, chances are they would be on the male variety—Botox or plastic surgery, anyone?
- On average, as of 2002, a woman makes $0.78 for every $1.00 that a man makes. This means that the usual weekly wage for female, full-time workers over the

197

age of sixteen is $530 a week, compared to an average of $680 for men. Female physicians have it worse than most professions: women docs are making $947 a week, while Dr. Man is making $1,626 a week (this is about 58 cents for female physicians for each dollar the male physician earns). Can we have a raise, please?[2]

- Women make up 51 percent of the United States population but only 14 percent of the United States Congress.[3]

- The amount of time allocated to household chores per workday by working mothers and fathers in dual-earner couples with children in 2002: women: 3 hours, men: 2 hours. The amount of time allocated to children per workday by working moms and dads in dual-earner couples: women: 3.5 hours, men 2.7 hours.[4] Nice to come home to extra dishes, childcare, and vacuuming after a hard day's work, right? It seems that neither parent is able to spend much time with their kids, either.

- Teachers call on girls less often than boys in math and science classes. Thanks for the encouragement.

Some Key Terms

✺ **Feminism** (coined in 1895 from the French *féminisme*): 1. the theory of the political, economic, and social equality of the sexes; 2. organized activity on behalf of women's rights and interests.

✺ **Grrrl:** Trading in wimpy "girl" connotations for the growling "grrrrrl," this word represents young feminists who are voicing their dissent with today's culture.

✺ **Misogyny:** Having or showing a hatred or distrust of women.

✺ **Patriarchy:** A system of male authority that oppresses women through its social, political, and economic institutions.

✺ **Sexism:** A term coined by feminists to describe social situations, both private and institutional, in which the idea that women are inferior to men prevails.

✺ **Womanism** (coined by Alice Walker and Chikwenye Okonjo Ogunyemi): An alternative term to feminism that broadens the focus from just gender to racial, cultural, sexual, national, economic, and political considerations.

- In more than three thousand films released between January 2000 and December 2004, fewer than four hundred were directed by women. When it comes to films, we are still missing in action.[5]

Given these less than cool facts, many women are continuing where their feminist sisters left off—uniting women with the beliefs that we must question sexual stereotypes and that opportunities should never, ever be denied to either men or women on the grounds of gender. As Betty Friedan, one of the mamas of contemporary feminism, said, "Women are people, in the fullest sense of the word, who must be free to move in society with all the privileges and opportunities and responsibilities that are their human right."

So what does it mean to be a feminist these days? Some of us think that feminism is about women being equal to men, better than men, or hating men. Others believe that feminism is not about men but about feeling empowered as females and reaching our full potential. No matter where we stand with feminism, diving into the issues is an adventure because we quickly discover that almost everyone has an opinion on the matter. What do you think? Read on.

I've always thought of myself as a feminist.

It means just being equal to men, on every level. Ever since I first heard the word, when I was a little kid, I thought of myself as a feminist. Maybe it's because my mom basically supports the whole family and my dad sits around. I've always known that women were strong.

—Lori, eighteen years old

I stand up for myself when I need to.

For example, if I feel like I'm being treated unfairly, I speak up. If my parents tell me I can't go out, I feel upset because I know boys get treated differently. I try to explain that I can take care of myself. Once, my nine-year-old male cousin was allowed to see Mortal Kombat *and I wasn't, even though I was five years older. My mom just said that's the way it is. I hate sexism—sometimes I feel like I could get a lot further if I was a guy.*

—Malika, fourteen years old

If a guy says, "Girls can't do that," I just think, "This guy is a fool."

I know girls can do whatever we want, but in my neighborhood, there is a lot of machismo and the guys I know think that girls aren't as good as they are. Sometimes I don't say anything because I don't want people to think I'm too aggressive. But my friend is a feminist, and she always says things back to the guys; she's more active. I guess I just figure they are stupid and it's not worth bothering.

—Marlena, sixteen years old

I think there should be equal rights for women, but I also like men to be manly—open doors, make decisions, and pay for meals.

When I think of feminists, I think of a girl who wants to be treated like a guy. I don't mind taking a step back and not shouting as loudly as men, and kind of letting them take the lead.

—Julie, eighteen years old

Boys might have more physical strength, but girls have more mental strength. At my school, the top ten students on the honor roll are girls.

I think girls are more motivated and work harder to prove the point that we can do as well or better than boys.

—Kelly, eighteen years old

I like to take advantage of being a girl.

I can act sweet in a way guys can't to get a favor done for me. I can get out of class because of a "woman's problem." Or if I get caught speeding, I can cry to get sympathy and avoid a ticket.

—Bea, sixteen years old

Feminism for me is being pro-women.

It doesn't come up with my group of friends. I am pro-women, but I don't identify with the part of the feminist movement that is anti-men. I don't think there should be conflict between men and women. I think the best thing would be if there wasn't a differentiation in terms of the work world . . . same as with the races.

—Maya, sixteen years old

Unplugged

The scalding look in her eyes
"You should wear feminine shoes,

you look like a truck driver"
"Let boys win or they won't like you"
"Suck in your tummy"
Made part of me die
Pushed a tough straw into my throat

That cut in her voice
"Why don't you spend more time on your hair?"
"Don't eat too much on a date"
Goes in deep. I'm not included
in her world, not quite a real girl
The clog in my throat grows more dense
It's harder to speak

For a time I manage to take my turn
Waiting for boys to call, pretending to lose
to their skill, having all the questions—
"What do you think, what do you like?"
But no answers

A moment comes I don't recognize
Myself in the mirror
I wonder again and again what's wrong with me?

Until I finally meet others
Who look beyond the mask and ask what I think
I pull a bamboo branch out from my stomach
Through my throat that's been clogging me up

I say I am real, I'm not just a part
Those shoes she urged make me wobble
And no one can know me

The words pour out and pull people I love around
Make me strong and whole.

—**Samantha Phillips**

The F-Word: Why Some of Us
Shun the Word "Feminist"

I don't think I should have to deny that I am a feminist.

People are afraid to say they are a feminist. They think feminists tell a guy who just says hello, "Go away, you chauvinist pig," and believe that all guys are scum. People are afraid that is what others will think of them if they say they are a feminist. I know some people think that about me because I have stickers on my locker from NARAL and stuff and I consider myself a feminist. Sometimes I do feel uncomfortable saying I am a feminist, but I hate that. I don't think I should have to deny that I am because of what people will think.

—Sinnead, sixteen years old

For many, "feminist" is a loaded label with which they'd rather not be identified. "Man hater," "rigid and politically correct," "in-your-face, sign-carrying women's libber," and "flat-chested and ugly" are just some of the ridiculous connotations associated with this innocent three-syllable word. Many of us wear our women-power t-shirts proudly and declare with assurance that of course we are feminists, how could we not want equal rights? Why is there so much disparity about embracing feminism? Now that there are women reclaiming the terms "bitch," "cunt," and "slut," surely we can reclaim the F-word and shout from our windows: "Yes, I'm a feminist."

A lot of the negative connotations attached to the word—baggage that persists even today—have to do with how certain folks and the media managed to turn feminism into a dirty word. Rather than listening to what feminists had to say, the popular media (surprise, surprise) focused on their looks, their mental health, their propensity (or lack thereof) to date men, and their feminine (or unfeminine) qualities. The following examples illustrate this:

- In the late 1800s, folks who didn't appreciate feminists' efforts to get women the vote asked, "Is it desirable to have women become masculine instead of retaining the characteristics of her own sex?"[6]

- In the early 1900s, many psychologists felt that feminism was associated with mental illness and tossed around the words "neurotic" and "penis envy" when describing feminists.[7]

- In 1947, doctors Ferdinand Lundberg and Marynia F. Farnham wrote a book called *Modern Woman: The Lost Sex* and stated that "feminism . . . was at its core a deep illness" and "the more educated the woman is, the greater chance there is of sexual disorder."

- In the early 1970s, Senator Jennings Randolph characterized the women's movement as "a small band of bra-less bubbleheads."[8] Phyllis Schlafly, the "let's kill the Equal Rights Amendment" crusader, chimed in with the remark, "Feminists just don't want to be nice. They want to be ugly."[9]

- In 1989, *Time* magazine wrote: "Hairy legs haunt the feminist movement" and announced that the movement was dead, kaput, done with.[10]

- In the 1990s, antifeminists like Camille Paglia and Christina Hoff Sommers reminded us that—yes—women are as effective as men at putting down feminists. These women accused feminists of being big whiners who create an atmosphere for male bashing, lie to get laws passed, and promote propaganda about female oppression. Paglia—perhaps the most in-your-face anti-feminist—represents this group well with her statement, "[Feminist scholars] can't think their way out of a wet paper bag."[11]

- In the early 2000s, writers like Dr. Laura Schlessinger *(The Proper Care and Feeding of Husbands)* and Laura Doyle *(The Surrendered Wife)* tell us that what women really want deep down is to nurture their hubbies. Boy, some of us have come a long way, baby!

In the face of all this, it takes guts to embrace the word and say, "Yes, I am a feminist." Oftentimes, we may feel compelled to provide some explanation, for example, that we appreciate men and for us the label does not mean "this" or "that." Or that we are more interested in girls being powerful and not taking a backseat than whether or not we use the F-word.

Equal pay for equal work.

Women can embrace the concepts of feminism but won't call themselves feminists because of the negative connotations. If you ask a lot of young women what the women's movement or feminism stands for, they would say, "Equal pay for equal work." And they believe that as females, they should be treated as equal citizens. But when you ask them if they consider themselves feminists, they say no. It's kind of hypocritical.

—Maddy, seventeen years old

I have a strong connection to the women's movement.

People think if you are a feminist then you hate men—it's such baloney. Girls I know are like, "I'm into women's rights and into equality—but I'm not a feminist," or "I'm into women's rights, but I don't hate men," all in the same breath. I have a problem with that. I think that it's a shame. I have a strong connection to the women's movement; I have since high school. People were like, "Why?" A lot of people put labels on feminists, which is like putting a label on the word "woman." People like that are not supportive at all; they are more anti-feminist.

When I first got involved in feminism, I knew what was running around in my parents' heads. I told them, "No, I'm not a lesbian." I think a lot of people assume things about your sexuality if you are pro-women. I understand that people don't want to be mislabeled (as a lesbian), but I think that shunning feminism is not going to fix that problem. I think if more women embrace the word and show they are individuals too, we can create a whole new meaning.

—Alix, eighteen years old

Feminism is such a taboo word!

People assume you are a dyke, you won't have children, and above all you hate men. I think it's changing a little, but I'm not sure how much. I am gay, but I knew about my sexuality way before I considered myself a feminist. I hate that some people think that my being a feminist made me gay.

—Kyra, fifteen years old

I don't necessarily say I'm a feminist, but my girlfriends and I stand up for each other and don't take any disrespect from boys.

We act tough and don't try to act or look stupid. I've noticed that the girls on TV shows are such bubbleheads, and I point that out—I wish there were stronger girls shown on TV. I see older girls who get into trouble when all they want to do is please a guy; they lose sight of themselves, and it's sad.

—Athena, fourteen years old

I think most women are feminists, they just don't want to say it.

There's nothing so special attached to it. It's basic: Women deserve respect for who they are. I think most people think that. They just don't say it, but I do.

—Talia, sixteen years old

The History of Feminism: The Road Toward Equality

Yes, I am a feminist.

My friends and I looked up "feminism" in the dictionary. It said that feminism was about political, economic, and social equality. When I saw that definition, I thought, yes, I am a feminist.

—Yun, seventeen years old

Before we come to any conclusion on whether or not we feel part of the feminist movement, or whether we even like the ideas of feminism, it helps to become familiar with what happened to get us where we are today. Learning about the women who took on unconventional roles and helped bring generations of women to new heights of accomplishment is inspiring. The following is a smattering about some of those brave women and some of the pivotal events in the history of the women's movement. Though this is an account of feminist history in the United States, keep in mind that there were and are feminist movements all over the globe. The American feminist movement is typically described in terms of "waves" of activity: The first wave concerned gaining the right to vote, and the second concerned women gaining equal rights in all respects. And the third wave—well, some would say it's too early to tell.

The First Wave: Demanding the Right to Vote

It's hard for us modern gals to believe that only a few generations ago, men felt that women's "delicate emotional equilibrium could be easily upset by a strain like voting."[12] Back then, the prediction was that disastrous results would occur if women were to vote because women could be easily "exploited." Opponents to universal suffrage even worried that women would skew election results by hiding extra ballots in the "voluminous sleeves" that were in fashion at the time.[13] The fight to get the vote was a long, hard, uphill battle—with rallies, hunger strikes, and boycotts. Suffragists even chained themselves to buildings and destroyed property (so much for the frail and dainty stereotype!). Here are some of the highlights:

Before Susan B. Anthony and our more modern sisters, there were some colonial gals eager to get women on more equal footing with their male counterparts. In the 1630s, Anne Hutchinson, a Massachusetts colonist, threatened to shake things up by preaching in public and encouraging other women "to be rather a husband than a wife." She was branded a heretic by the Puritans and banished from the

Pandora's Pages

Feminism is a dynamic and diverse movement. Take a look at this selection of feminist classics:

Nonfiction

Ain't I a Woman: Black Women and Feminism by bell hooks, Boston: South End Press, 1981.

The American Women's Almanac: An Inspiring and Irreverent Women's History by Louise Bernikow (in association with the National Women's History Project), New York: Berkley Books, 1997.

Backlash: The Undeclared War Against American Women by Susan Faludi, New York: Crown Books, 1991.

The Feminine Mystique by Betty Friedan, New York: W. W. Norton, 2001.

Home Girls: A Black Feminist Anthology edited by Barbara Smith, New Brunswick, NJ: Rutgers University Press, 2000.

In Search of Our Mothers' Gardens: Womanist Prose by Alice Walker, New York: Harcourt Brace, 2004.

No More Nice Girls: Countercultural Essays by Ellen Willis, Hanover, NH: Wesleyan University Press, 1992.

Outrageous Acts and Everyday Rebellions by Gloria Steinem, New York: Henry Holt, 1995.

A Room of One's Own by Virginia Woolf, New York: Harcourt Brace, 1991.

The Second Sex by Simone de Beauvoir, New York: Alfred A. Knopf, 1993.

Sexual Politics by Kate Millett, Garden City, NY: Simon & Schuster, 1990.

Sister Outsider: Essays and Speeches by Audre Lorde, Trumansburg, NY: Crossing Press, 1984.

Sisterhood Is Powerful: An Anthology of Writings from the Women's Liberation Movement edited by Robin Morgan, New York: Random House, 1970.

This Bridge Called My Back: Writings by Radical Women of Color edited by
  Gloria Anzaldúa and Cherríe Moraga, Berkeley, CA: Third Woman Press,
  2002.

Where the Girls Are: Growing Up Female with the Mass Media by Susan J.
  Douglas, New York: Times Books, 1994.

Women, Race, and Class by Angela Y. Davis, New York: Vintage Books, 1983.

Autobiography and Memoir

Borderlands/La Frontera: The New Mestiza by Gloria Anzaldúa, San Francisco:
  Aunt Lute Books, 1999.

I Know Why the Caged Bird Sings by Maya Angelou, New York: Random House,
  2002.

I, Rigoberta Menchú: An Indian Woman in Guatemala by Elisabeth Burgos-
  Debray, Rigoberta Menchú and Ann Wright, London: Verso Books, 1984.

The Woman Warrior: Memoirs of a Girlhood Among Ghosts by Maxine Hong
  Kingston, New York: Vintage International, 1989.

Fiction and Poetry

The Awakening by Kate Chopin, New York: Oxford University Press, 2000.

The Bluest Eye by Toni Morrison, New York: Plume, 1994.

The Fact of a Doorframe: Poems Selected and New 1950–1984 by Adrienne
  Rich, New York: W. W. Norton, 1984.

The Handmaid's Tale by Margaret Atwood, Boston: Houghton Mifflin, 1986.

The Moon Is Always Female: Poems by Marge Piercy, New York: Knopf, 1980.

My Antonia by Willa Cather, New York: Modern Library, 1996.

Their Eyes Were Watching God by Zora Neale Hurston, New York:
  HarperCollins, 2000.

The Yellow Wallpaper by Charlotte Perkins Gilman, Boston: Bedford Books,
  1998.

colony![14] And in 1776, Abigail Adams warned her husband and future president, John, "If particular care and attention is not paid to the Ladies, we are determined to form a Rebellion and will not hold ourselves bound by any Laws in which we have no voice, or Representation."[15] You go, Abby!

Effective, organized action didn't come until the 1800s. At that time, women were becoming better educated, which naturally led some to think, "Hey, why do the boys get all the power?" Women became more involved in social issues, and there was a gradual emergence of women's groups devoted to achieving equal rights with men.

In 1848, Elizabeth Cady Stanton and Lucretia Coffin Mott organized a women's rights convention, which three hundred women attended. The event is generally considered the beginning of the modern feminist movement. The convention adopted Stanton's "Declaration of Sentiments," which asserted that all men and women were created equal. These way-hip women called for full legal, social, and political equality with men, along with increased educational and professional opportunities. Most important, though, was the demand for the right to vote—formally launching the American campaign for women's suffrage. For the next several years, women activists, now known as "suffragists," sponsored similar conventions.

In 1851, Sojourner Truth gave her famous "Ain't I a woman?" speech at an Ohio women's rights convention. Truth, born into slavery, was a human rights advocate who spoke out about the oppression of both blacks and women. Savvy Sojourner's honest words attacked the suffragist movement for its racism. Her words live on today and encourage us to fight against the stupidity of those who would keep others down. At the 1851 convention, she reportedly said the following in reply to several men's opinions on the inferiority of women. She was pointing out that as a black woman, she received different treatment than white women—showing that the first-wave feminists were not addressing issues relevant to black women's lives:

That man over there says that women need to be helped into carriages, and lifted over ditches, and to have the best place everywhere. Nobody ever helps me into carriages, or over mud-puddles, or gives me any best place! And ain't I a woman?

In the last half of the nineteenth century, Susan B. Anthony and other suffragists brought the protest for equal rights to new heights. Sophisticated Susan fought for equal treatment starting at a young age, when she insisted that her male teacher should teach her, as well as the boys, how to do long division. Susan was stubborn in her fight for women's right to vote and in 1871 was arrested and fined one hundred dollars for registering herself and fifteen other women to vote. Our hats are off to sister Susan for taking such a strong stand.

Slowly but surely, the country started coming to its senses. In 1869, Wyoming let women have some political muscle: As a territory, it granted them the right to vote, and it continued this practice when it became a state in 1890. Other states followed suit. Finally, in 1919, Congress approved the Nineteenth Amendment to the U.S. Constitution: "The right of citizens of the United States to vote shall not be denied or abridged by the United States or any State on account of sex." Over a year later, the required thirty-six states had ratified the amendment and it became law. Since then, women have been voting and not suffering from any strain, despite what some had predicted.

Having attained its goal—women's right to vote—the feminist movement dwindled in both size and energy over the next few decades. But during this time, women's growing role in the workplace was creating the groundwork for a second wave of feminist action.

> **Did you know?** Way back in 1872, Victoria Woodhull, a stockbroker, publisher, and protégé of Cornelius Vanderbilt, ran for president of the United States on the Equal Rights Party ticket. [16]

The Second Wave: The Personal Is Political

I think feminism means that you think women are equal to men.
Everyone is equal; one sex shouldn't be on a platform above another. We should get paid the same amount for the same job. My friends all think feminism is fine, and the guys I know are all used to it.
                                                        —Mandee, sixteen years old

The slogan for the second wave of feminism was "The Personal Is Political" because it brought attention to the fact that how women are treated on a personal level (as workers, moms, and lovers) is significant on a wider political scale. This wave focused on social problems like equal opportunity, equal pay, abortion rights, domestic violence, and rape. Witty slogans on bumper stickers, signs, and t-shirts expressed the unrest: "Sink into his arms and soon your arms will be in his sink." The second wave reached

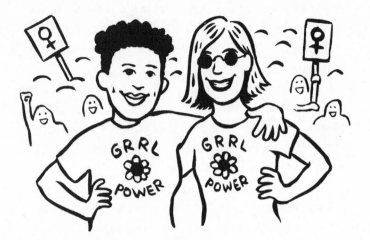

its height in the late 1960s and 1970s, when sisters united to bring these issues to the public eye and demanded change. Here's a quick rundown of second-wave events:

The Postwar Backlash
During World War II, while the boys were off fighting in Europe and the South Pacific, six million women went to work for the first time, mostly in factory and clerical jobs in war-related industries. After the war, there was a surge of anti-feminism throughout the country. In the 1950s, many women left jobs to be stay-at-home moms because that was thought to be their "proper place." This era was full of advertisements and television shows depicting the happy housewife, fulfilled by baking cookies for the kids and buying new appliances. Prominent psychologists told women that their essential function was to be a submissive and fertile wife.

The Sixties
In the 1960s, the narrow view of the feminine role became harder and harder for women to swallow. In 1963, Betty Friedan published *The Feminine Mystique*, which blew the top off the myth of the blissed-out housewife. Brilliant Betty relieved thousands of women by noting that sometimes cleaning the house and doing the laundry were less than fulfilling. She opened the way for women to explore fulfillment outside of the role of wife and mother and helped start the National Organization for Women in 1966. This group continues to fight for increased political representation for women, equal rights in employment and education, and women's reproductive rights.

Also in 1963, President John F. Kennedy's Commission on the Status of Women released a report documenting widespread sexism. In 1964, the Equal Pay Act was passed, along with the Civil Rights Act, which prohibited discrimination on the basis of sex, race, religion, and national origin.

In 1968, a group of brave and with-it women, led by Robin Morgan, protested the Miss America Pageant in Atlantic City by placing a crown on a sheep to illustrate that beauty pageants judge women "like animals at a county fair." They chanted, "Atlantic City is a town with class. They raise your morals and judge your ass."

The Seventies

In the early 1970s, women like Gloria Steinem helped bring feminism to the main-stream. Groovy Gloria had a major influence in legalizing abortion—sharing her per-sonal experience with an illegal abortion and coining the term "reproductive freedom." Gloria also helped launch *Ms.* in 1972—a newsmagazine dedicated to cov-ering women's movements around the world—with the hope of unifying feminists and promoting sisterhood. Gloria also pleased the media because she was "pretty." More people could swallow her pro-feminist statements because, hey, she looked good enough to get a guy *and* she was a feminist.

Building on momentum that had been increasing for some time, several organi-zations formed to support and strengthen African American feminists' voices and call for an end to all faces of oppression. In 1973, the National Black Feminist Organization was founded in New York and the Black Women Organized for Action Group was formed in San Francisco. In 1974, the Combahee River Collective was initiated, with the following declaration: "We see Black feminism as the logical political movement to combat the manifold and simultaneous oppressions that all women of color face."[17]

In 1974, the Mexican American Women's National Association was formed to provide a voice for Mexican American women at national, state, and local levels. Also in the 1970s, "radical feminists" contributed to the emerging feminist theory, making us take a second, and third, look at how patriarchy has shaped our society. Kate Millett wrote *Sexual Politics,* a bestseller and the most in-demand book in the 1970s feminist movement. People were stirred up by cutting-edge Kate's ideas that marriage was a financial arrangement in which men win and women lose. The media loved calling Kate an ugly, man-hating woman who turned feminist only because she was rejected by men one too many times. Mary Daly, who wrote *Gyn/Ecology: The Metaethics of Radical Feminism* in 1978, thought that women bought "truths" written by men—like the Bible, law, and science—hook, line, and sinker and were thus "moronized." She wrote, "Patriarchy has stolen our cosmos and returned it in the form of *Cosmopolitan* magazine and cosmetics." Modern Mary concluded that we needed to invent ourselves without thinking about men's ideology—in order to re-create ourselves and take care of the earth.

The seventies were full of women speaking out, just as Helen Reddy sang out:

> I am woman, hear me roar
> In numbers too big to ignore
> And I know too much to go back, to pretend
> 'Cause I've heard it all before
> And I've been down there on the floor
> No one's ever gonna keep me down again . . .
>
> If I have to, I can do anything
> I am strong, I am invincible
> I am woman . . .
>
> **–Helen Reddy, "I Am Woman,"** *Lust for Life*

The Eighties

While the pendulum was starting to swing back against feminism and some were saying that women had come far enough, others kept the fight for equality active in the early eighties. Some new inspirational feminist writings appeared; *All the Women Are White, All the Blacks Are Men, But Some of Us are Brave: Black Women's Studies*, edited by Gloria T. Hull, Patricia Bell Scott, and Barbara Smith, was published in 1982; *Sister Outsider: Essays and Speeches*, by Audre Lorde, was published in 1984. This collection of Lorde's writing addressed issues such as gender, sexism, race, racism, and social class. She wrote: "Women of today are still being called upon to stretch across the gap of male ignorance and to educate men as to our existence and our needs. This is an old and primary tool of all oppressors to keep the oppressed occupied with the master's concerns."

The ERA Saga

The saga of the Equal Rights Amendment (ERA) spanned both the first and second waves of the feminist movement. The first Equal Rights Amendment was introduced to Congress in 1923 by the National Woman's Party (founded in 1916). In 1943, Senator Hattie Caraway became the first woman in Congress to sponsor the ERA, which called for a ratification of the simple statement: "Equality of rights under the law shall not be denied or abridged by the United States or by any State on account of sex." The ERA was essentially a clarification that, yup, women are actually people too and deserve guaranteed equal rights. In 1946, the Senate voted on the ERA, but it was defeated thirty-eight to thirty-five. Then, in 1967, the newly formed National Organization for Women called for the immediate passage of the ERA. By 1972, both the House and the Senate had passed the ERA. But for the ERA to become law, it needed the states' approval, and by 1982, it was defeated by a lack of just three states.

What went wrong? The ERA, a basic statement that obviously seems to be a good thing, managed to make quite a commotion. It was staunchly opposed by folks like Phyllis Schlafly, whose 1972 "Stop the ERA" and subsequent campaigns got a lot of attention and effectively helped prevent the ERA from passing. Fuming Phyllis used the negative stereotypes of feminists for all they were worth, with biting comments like, "Feminists are a bunch of bitter women seeking a constitutional cure for their personal problems."[18] Phyllis was not a very helpful sister, to say the least! Other women were concerned that there was too much E in the ERA and that this would hurt women in situations like the military draft, divorce and child custody cases, and maternity leave. More than seventy years after its introduction, the ERA is still not law. Today, many groups continue to fight and stand for the equal rights of women everywhere. Along with the ERA, there are important issues to promote: human rights (there are countries where women are denied the right to vote, endure genital mutilation, have little or no legal recourse, and do not have equal access to education); abortion rights; and encouraging more women to take on political and leadership roles.

We haven't reached equality yet. It may even be generations away.

There are little subtle everyday things, like how men act toward women or how commercials use sexy women to sell cars. Sometimes I think we are even moving in the wrong direction.

—Mica, eighteen years old

Girls are a lot stronger now than they used to be—because feminists spoke out.

They brought things like sexual harassment to everyone's attention. They protested and kept pushing the idea that things weren't acceptable. We wouldn't be where we are today. Now a girl won't listen to a guy who says he's better than her.

—Jessica, sixteen years old

Women of Color and Feminism: Ending Oppression on All Fronts

> I never felt myself—in my experience as a rural Black person—
> included in the first feminist books I read, works like The
> *Feminine Mystique* and *Born Female*.... Since so many of the
> early feminist books really reflected a certain type of white bour-
> geois sensibility, this work did not touch many Black women
> deeply; not because we did not recognize the common experi-
> ences women share, but because those commonalities were
> mediated by profound differences in our realities created by
> the politics of race and class.
>
> —**bell hooks**, *Teaching to Transgress*

Recent Firsts for Women

It is amazing how many firsts for women have taken place in our lifetime. Over the past three decades, women have made huge gains and won many victories. We are still breaking new ground:

1976 Barbara Walters becomes the first woman to anchor a network evening newscast.

1978 National Aeronautics and Space Administration (NASA) accepts women for astronaut training.

1981 Sandra Day O'Connor is the first woman to sit on the Supreme Court (in 1993 she is joined by Ruth Bader Ginsburg).

1981 Barbara Hutchinson is the first black woman to be a member of the AFL-CIO executive council.

1982 Jeane Jordan Kirkpatrick is the first woman to represent the United States as permanent ambassador to the United Nations.

1983 Sally K. Ride is the first American woman in space.

I think black women are often concerned with different issues than white women.

Like we are thinking about why so many black men are in jail. And we have a lot of issues on the home front, like having more positive black role models for our kids. I think of white feminists as concerned about job equality and politics, topics that I'm not thinking much about.

—Yolanda, eighteen years old

African American, Asian American, Latina, and Native American women have criticized and ultimately strengthened the feminist movement by bringing multiracial viewpoints to the struggle and broadening the movement's scope. These perspectives have helped the movement evolve toward an understanding that the women's struggle for rights is within a racist society and that all oppression needs to be

1984 Geraldine Ferraro is the first female vice-presidential candidate of a major political party.

1985 Wilma Mankiller becomes the first woman principal chief of the Cherokee Nation.

1989 Dr. Antonia C. Novello is the first female surgeon general.

1993 Janet Reno is the first female attorney general, and Toni Morrison is the first African American woman to win the Nobel prize for literature.

1994 Shannon Faulkner becomes the first woman to attend the all-male Citadel, a prestigious military training institute.

1997 Madeleine Albright is the first female Secretary of State.

2000 Hillary Rodham Clinton is the first wife of a president to run for national office. Not only does she run, but she wins and becomes a U.S. senator, representing New York State.

2001 Condoleezza Rice becomes the first female National Security Advisor to the president of the United States.

2004 On a global note, in 2004 Wangari Maathai from Kenya became the first African woman to win a Nobel Peace Prize.

dismantled in unison. For example, in 1895, one hundred African American women met in Boston under the guidance of Josephine St. Pierre Ruffin to create the National Federation of Afro-American Women. The group was formed in reaction to sexism and racism and because the existing feminist groups, which were led by white women, were only concerned with upper-middle-class issues. They wanted to

Feminists Organize

Let your voice be heard—stand up for the causes you believe in:

Center for Women's Global Leadership
Douglass College, Rutgers University
160 Ryders Land
New Brunswick, NJ 08901
phone: (732) 932-8782
website: www.cwgl.rutgers.edu

The Eleanor Roosevelt Center at Val-Kill
PO Box 255
Hyde Park, NY 12538
phone: (845) 229-5302
website: www.ervk.org

Feminist Majority Foundation
1600 Wilson Boulevard, Suite 801
Arlington, VA 22209
phone: (703) 522-2214
website: www.feminist.org

Girls, Inc. (National Office)
120 Wall Street
New York, NY 10005
phone: (212) 509-2000
website: www.girlsinc.org

National Organization for Women
1000 16th Street NW, Suite 700
Washington, D.C. 20036
phone: (202) 331-0066
website: www.now.org

Third Wave Foundation
511 W. 25th Street, Suite 301
New York, NY 10001
phone: (212) 675-0700
website: www.thirdwave
foundation.org

The Woodhull Institute
770 Broadway, 2nd Floor
New York, NY 10003
phone: (646) 495-6060
website: www.woodhull.org

defend black women and men from racism—particularly some of the extreme violence they witnessed, including lynchings. The group fought for its own issues but also eventually came together with the white suffragists to rally for the right of women to vote as a means toward women's equality.

Women of color continued to blaze trails during feminism's second wave. In the 1970s, while the civil rights movement was in full swing, women of color brought feminism to task by alerting both movements that sexism and racism had to be fought together—that it's simply not possible to uproot them individually, not only because women come in all races but because racism and sexism reinforce each other. Angela Davis, an African American feminist leader, supported socialist reform as a means to attaining the goals of feminism. Activist Angela felt that after a political revolution, a revolution in women's roles would follow. (After all, the economic class system is what historically has given men economic and political power.)

Here are a few highlights of some of the actions taken by women of color in the feminist movement.

- The Mexican American Women's National Association was formed in 1974 and is now is a large national Latina organization—expanding into all corners of the political, social, and professional landscape.
- In 1981, Chicana feminists Gloria Anzaldua and Cherrie Moraga co-edited *This Bridge Called My Back: Writings by Radical Women of Color*. When their publisher went out of business, Moraga co-founded Kitchen Table/Women of Color Press and kept *This Bridge Called My Back* in print. The book won praise and readership nationwide, and both Moraga and Anzaldua went on to be highly regarded writers.
- Asian Women United of California published *Making Waves: An Anthology of Writings by and about Asian American Women* in 1989, breaking stereotypes and giving voice to Asian women writers. *Making More Waves: New Writing by Asian American Women* was published in 1997.
- African American writer, feminist, and professor bell hooks has contributed much to today's multicultural literature with books like *Ain't I a Woman: Black Women and Feminism, Yearning: Race, Gender, and Cultural Politics, and Teaching to Transgress: Education As the Practice of Freedom*. Her contributions highlight the specific issues faced by being a woman of color and a feminist.

Today's young women find their place where they feel strongest and most comfortable—for some feminism hits home, for others it seems lacking.

Being black, I hear the word feminism and I think of white women who have tea parties.

I just don't identify with the word at all. At the same time, I admire strong black women like Queen Latifah—she's a great role model. I'm all for women being strong.

—Kenia, seventeen years old

Feminism is universal—it's not just for one race or another.

Women of all races and classes can unite and fight if they see injustice in the world. I'm proud to be a woman, and I'm proud of my color. Both contribute to who I am.

—Malika, fourteen years old

My friends and I are all feminists, which for me means combating the stereotype of the weak, passive Asian woman.

I really speak my mind, and I tell my boyfriend what I think and expect him to respect my opinions. I feel my identity as a feminist is mainly on a personal level. I'm not so active in the bigger community because I have to forge my way at home as a strong Asian woman.

—Yun, seventeen years old

Feminism Today: Are We Riding a Third Wave?

Jigsaw Jigsaw youth
We know there's not
one way
one light
one stupid truth

don't fit yr definitions
won't meet yr demands
not into
win/lose reality
won't fit in with
your plan

—Bikini Kill, "Jigsaw Youth," *Bikini Kill*

So where is feminism today? We can major in women's studies and are told we can be anything we want, but some of us strongly feel there is still work to be done for women to reach their fullest potential: We're fed up with feeling oppressed by the beauty and fashion culture, being told we have to be thin to win, and hearing myths about our sexuality. We are also overwhelmed by the pressure to have a fabulous career while being the world's best mom and homemaker. Many of our contemporaries are working hard to make women's voices and concerns heard—and they are not all doing it in one way. The following is a list of diva organizations, resources, and movements that are dedicated to raising consciousness about where girls and women are today:

Riot Grrrls

An attitude that emerged in the early 1990s out of the male-dominated punk music scene. Grrrls like Kathleen Hanna of Bikini Kill and Allison Wolfe of Bratmobile rejected the mainstream media as not reflecting young women's concerns. Through their music and writing, Riot Grrrls helped create an atmosphere where girls could voice their frustrations and give free rein to their creativity. Awesome music and writing flourished, expressing countercultural ideas on a very personal level about fat oppression, sexism, and the media's insane beauty standards. Key to the Riot Grrrl movement is girls supporting each other and fighting the stereotype of female backstabbing and cattiness.

Guerrilla Girls

In the 1980s, a group of women decided to get vocal about the male-dominated art world. Anonymous behind furry gorilla masks, they use humor to bring folks' attention to the crazy biases against women artists and artists of color and to prove that, yes, feminists have a sense of humor! They create posters like the following:

Q: Do women have to be naked to get into the Metropolitan Museum?

A: Less than 5 percent of the artists in the Museum Art sections are women, but 85 percent of the nudes are female.

The Guerrilla Girls are a powerful inspiration for us to be creative with our activism and not be afraid to take a stand for change. They now have a political theater group and perform plays to bring feminist issues to the forefront—all the while maintaining a great sense of humor.

Want to be a Guerrilla Girl? Surf to their internet address at www.guerillagirls.com or read one of their books: *Confessions of the Guerrilla Girls* (HarperCollins, 1995), *The Guerrilla Girls' Bedside Companion to the History of Western Art* (Viking, 1998), and *Bitches, Bimbos and Ballbreakers: The Guerilla Girls' Illustrated Guide to Female Stereotypes* (Penguin Books, 2003).

Third Wave Foundation

In 1992, Rebecca Walker and Shannon Liss, both in their early twenties, co-founded the Third Wave Direct Action Corporation to encourage young women to be feminist leaders and activists. With support from some second-wavers like Gloria Steinem, the third wave movement took off with a bang. In 1997, Third Wave Direct Action Corporation became the Third Wave Foundation, a thriving nonprofit that, today, is the only activist philanthropic organization in the United States for young women between the ages of fifteen and thirty. The Third Wave Foundation informs and empowers young feminist activists through its network, public education campaigns, and grant-giving.

To gain some sisterly support (including possible financial support) for your feminist activities, check them out at www.thirdwavefoundation.org; you can also write to them at 511 W 25th Street, Suite 301, New York, NY 10001, or call (212) 675-0700.

Ending Violence: CODEPINK and Vagina Warriors

There are courageous women who are making waves and creating social change by gathering women together and making a strong, female stand for peace and the end of violence . . . now! Here are two organizations at the forefront of this movement.

CODEPINK

Medea Benjamin, Starhawk, Jodie Evans, Diane Wilson, and approximately one hundred other women kicked off CODEPINK on November 17, 2002, as a response to the buildup toward war in Iraq. In their own words, CODEPINK is "a women ini-tiated grassroots peace and social justice movement that seeks positive social change through proactive, creative protest and non-violent direct action." These ladies make themselves known by showing up in pink to protest for peace and say what's on their minds (they've been seen on CNN, in *The New York Times*, and on camera at the 2004 Republican Convention). If we are interested in helping to cre-ate social change and ready to get out there and give peace a chance, we should check this organization out. They offer events, local chapters, and training camps for activists.

Write to CODEPINK at 2010 Linden Avenue, Venice, CA 90291, give them a call at (310) 827-4320, or check them out on the web at www.codepink4peace.org.

Vagina Warriors

Eve Ensler wrote a play in 1994 that became a global movement. *The Vagina Monologues* is based on Eve's interviews with more than two hundred women and celebrates women's sexuality and strength. Vaginas were placed in the spotlight, and the world couldn't get enough: The play has been translated into more than thirty-five languages and is running in theaters all over the world. The success of this play birthed V-Day, a nonprofit that is committed to ending violence against women and girls everywhere. V-Day supports anti-violence organizations through-out the world, helping them to continue and expand their core work on the ground, while drawing public attention to the larger fight to stop worldwide violence (including rape, battery, incest, female genital mutilation, and sexual slavery) against women and girls.

If we are interested in attending a V-Day event, joining a V-Campaign, or taking on a V-Activity, we can check out www.vday.org or call (212) 645-8329.

Girls should just be individuals and think for themselves.

The problem with some women's groups is they tell you how you have to be, like you can't care about your appearance or shave your legs. And that becomes oppressing. Feminism should listen to everyone's voices. You should worry about who you are and what you want—it's individualism, not feminism. My role model is myself—I love making mistakes and learning. Nobody else is me. I know what I've been through to get equality.

—Kiwessa, eighteen years old

Riot Grrrls and the whole punk thing was good because they made people listen, and they kept saying, "Don't ignore us." I got into the scene two years ago.

There were twenty of us, and one girl was the leader. She was off-the-wall and wanted chicks to run things. This experience opened me up to feeling powerful as a girl.

—Hailey, seventeen years old

There's a danger when women activists become more mainstream.

They turn into cliques of giggling girls, not using their minds to change things or make a difference. They use catch phrases like "revolution now," but there's no action.

—Gwenn, seventeen years old

Feminism, Grrrl Style

Feminism continues to evolve, and young women face different issues than our mothers did. Check out some writing that is relevant to our current generation of feminists:

Boundaries of Her Body: The Troubling History of Women's Rights in America by Debran Rowland, Naperville, IL: Sphinx Publishing Inc., 2004.

Colonize This! Young Women of Color on Today's Feminism edited by Daisy Hernandez and Bushra Rehman, Emeryville, CA: Seal Press, 2002.

Cunt: A Declaration of Independence by Inga Muscio, Emeryville, CA: Seal Press, 2002.

The F-Word: Feminism in Jeopardy by Kristin Rowe-Finkbeiner, Emeryville, CA: Seal Press, 2004.

Feminism is for Everybody: Passionate Politics by bell hooks, Cambridge, MA: South End Press, 2000.

Girl Power: Young Women Speak Out by Hillary Carlip, New York: Warner Books, 1995.

GirlWise: How to Be Confident, Capable, Cool, and in Control by Julia Devillers, Roseville, CA: Prima Pub, 2002.

Creating Tomorrow's Leaders . . .
And Let's Make It a Woman This Time

There are a lot of people who are tired of always having men in the driver's seat when it comes to politics and foreign affairs. The statistics say it all:

- The United States has never had a woman in the office of the vice president or president (Great Britain and India are among the nations that are way ahead of us on this).
- If Congress and state governorships are the pipelines to the presidency, then those lines are only sprinkled with women—with 86 percent of congressional seats and 84 percent of governorships held by men.[19]

Kiss My Tiara: How to Rule the World as a Smartmouth Goddess by Susan Jane Gilman, New York: Warner Books, 2001.

Listen Up: Voices from the Next Feminist Generation edited by Barbara Findlen, Seattle: Seal Press, 2001.

Manifesta: Young Women, Feminism and the Future by Jennifer Baumgardner and Amy Richards, New York: Farrar Straus & Giroux, 2000.

Ophelia Speaks: Adolescent Girls Write about Their Search for Self edited by Sara Shandler, New York: HarperPerennial, 1999.

Present Tense: Writing and Art by Young Women edited by Micki Reaman et al., Corvalis, OR: Calyx Books, 1996.

Sugar in the Raw: Voices of Young Black Girls in America edited by Rebecca Carroll, New York: Crown,1997.

Third Wave Agenda: Being Feminist, Doing Feminism edited by Leslie Heywood and Jennifer Drake, Minneapolis: University of Minnesota Press, 1997.

To Be Real: Telling the Truth and Changing the Face of Feminism edited by Rebecca Walker, New York: Anchor Books, 1995.

Yell-Oh Girls!: Emerging Voices Explore Culture, Identity, and Growing Up Asian American edited by Vickie Nam, New York: Quill, 2001.

Yentl's Revenge: The Next Wave of Jewish Feminism edited by Danya Ruttenberg, Seattle: Seal Press, 2001.

- Women comprise only 13 percent of the Senate and 14 percent of the House of Representatives.
- Women represent only 11 percent of all guests on Sunday morning political talk shows.
- Young women, as well as young men, see politics as something "old white men" do. Or, they believe that "old white men" are only driven by money and are largely corrupt.[20]

Interested in changing the stats and seeing a woman in the Oval Office (one who is not serving the coffee)? The White House Project is a non-profit group dedicated to fostering the entry of women into positions of leadership, including the presidency. Write to The White House Project at 110 Wall Street, 2nd Floor, New York, NY 10005, call (212) 785-6001, or read up on the group at www.thewhitehouseproject.org.

Taking Our Rants and Ideas Public: Zines and Blogs

Zines

> I will always remain grateful to Grrl punk and zine culture for
> teaching me to speak the truth, love my freakishness, and make
> my own freedom. It started me on the journey.[21]
>
> **–Leah Lilith Albrecht-Samarasinha, editor of the zines**
> ***Patti Smith* and *Sticks and Stones***

Zines (or their electronic counterparts, e-zines) and blogs are ways that we can get our opinions, attitudes, and creative thoughts out to a community of like-minded sisters. Zines became hot in the mid-eighties as "do it yourself" publications that express the authors' often countercultural and politically cutting-edge opinions. Originally, they were typed, photocopied, and distributed locally but nowadays, if we have something to say, we can publish an e-zine online and have an audience of thousands without any photocopying or mailing expenses. There's a zine to appeal to almost everyone. Some great ones for girls include *I'm So Fucking Beautiful, Asian Girls Are Rad,* and *Fat!So?*

Check out www.zinebook.com for lots of information, including places that are storing archives of past zines and tips on how to build an e-zine. Also check out *A Girl's Guide to Taking Over the World: Writings from the Girl Zine Revolution* edited by Karen Green and Tristan Taormino (St. Martin's, 1997).

Blogs

> A blog is a personal diary. A daily pulpit. A collaborative space.
> A political soapbox. A breaking-news outlet. A collection of
> links. Your own private thoughts. Memos to the world. Your blog
> is whatever you want it to be. There are millions of them, in all
> shapes and sizes, and there are no real rules.
>
> **– www.bloggers.com**

A blog is a personal website that is updated frequently with diary-type entries as well as links, photos, and anything else we'd like to add to it. The latest entry is seen first, and the older items flow down the page or are archived and available through links. Blogs are great for self-expression, as a free-flow creative outlet, and for creating a movement of one or many. They can address a single topic or cover a hodgepodge of things. Blogs (based on the phrase "web log") are unique to the internet and require access to a computer and software for creating the webpage.

To set your thoughts free on the world or see how others are doing so, check out www.bloggers.com, a great resource on everything blog, including free software for creating your own. Also, check out www.bust.com for girl blog and journal links, and www.globeblogs.com, where we can register our blog and search for blogs from around the world.

Finding Our Own Brand of Feminism

> There are an infinite number of moments and experiences that
> make up female empowerment.
>
> **–Rebecca Walker,**
> **from the introduction of**
> ***To Be Real: Telling the Truth and Changing the Face of Feminism***

Each generation has an opportunity to define feminism for itself. And even within one generation, we don't all want the same thing or express ourselves in the same way (that would make the planet a boring place to live, no?). Within the world of feminism, we can find liberal feminists, radical feminists, conservative feminists, socialist feminists, lesbian feminists, spiritual feminists, ecofeminists, vegetarian feminists, superstar feminists, and on and on. Some of us find our own brand of womanhood without any feminist label. Although there is a lot of diversity in sisterhood, remembering our common ground is also key to moving forward on the road to empowerment.

Feminism has had a strong influence on global politics, life, and culture. We are one of the first generations to grow up expecting to be treated on equal terms with men. With a wealth of opportunities and many powerful role models, we now have a chance to build on what's already been put in place and evolve in a way that truly enlivens us. We can choose to embrace the term "feminist"—wanting equal rights for women—and not let the word be further maligned.

Some of us are on an ardent quest to find new ground—to be critical and informed consumers of the media, to throw away what doesn't work for us, and to

Get Involved

Once we have the right to vote at age eighteen, we can take every opportunity to get out and have our voices heard at the ballot box—after all, politics is not a spectator sport. Check out www.youthvote.com, a nonpartisan website designed to get young people involved in politics. Also, www.punkvoter.com is a motivating website where punk bands, musicians, and record labels have built a coalition to educate, register, and mobilize progressive voters.

Here are some other web links that transform apathy into enthusiasm and motivation:

Women & Leadership

Gender Gap
www.gendergap.com

Women Leaders Online
www.wlo.org

Institute for Women's Leadership
at Rutgers University
iwl.rutgers.edu

Institute for Women's Leadership
www.womensleadership.com

Center for Policy Alternatives
www.stateaction.org

Women & Politics

Center for American Women
and Politics
www.cawp.rutgers.edu

Women and Politics Institute
www.american.edu/oconnor/wandp/

League of Women Voters Democracy
Net
www.dnet.org

create new leaps in consciousness—so that we and our sisters can be the strongest, most creative, and most powerful females possible. Grrrl power, the web and zine scenes, vagina warriors, and cutting-edge artists are giving us liberating role models and helping to create new images of women. Where we feel the most empowered is up to us—we can be cool, savvy, funny, and politically active, while creating our own firsts for women.

I would define feminism as looking at the world with acceptance of what people do.

It's looking at people as individuals rather than statistics or only seeing their

National Foundation for Women Legislators
www.womenlegislators.org

National Women's Political Caucus
www.nwpc.org

Women's Campaign Fund
www.wcfonline.org

Women's Campaign Research Fund
www.womenlead.org

Women's Campaign School at Yale University
www.wcsyale.org

Women Matter
www.womenmatter.com

League of Women Voters
www.lwv.org

Women and Public Policy Program
www.ksg.harvard.edu/wappp/

Center for Women in Politics & Public Policy at University of Massachusetts Boston
www.mccormack.umb.edu/cwppp/

Women and Politics:
A Global Perspective
www.auburn.edu/outreach/womenandpolitics

Women in the News

The News We Can Use
www.newswecanuse.com
To create changes in leadership, it helps to know what's shaking. The News We Can Use site highlights women-centered headlines and stories from major and alternative media sources, and covers politics, health, the workplace, reproductive rights, and more. It's an easy way for us to stay abreast of women who are movin' and groovin'.

gender. And I think people really lose sight of that when they see the word "feminism." For a lot of people, abortion is the automatic litmus test for feminism. I think we need to separate the issues. There's a group called Feminists for Life, and they are pretty much the same as me except when it comes to abortion. We need to look for the common ground.

—Callie, fifteen years old

Instead of being a feminist, I say I'm an individual.

It's important to think for yourself. People don't like to think for themselves, because it's easier to follow society's assumptions and stereotypes. I don't listen to TV; I decide who I want to be. Stereotypes about males and females are awful. I have more "masculinity" than some guys I know. Everyone has some "masculinity" and some "femininity," and every individual should have a choice about who they are.

—Zara, eighteen years old

People need to accept that women will fight for equality, instead of dismissing women activists as having a man-hating lesbian agenda.

A lot of people remember the feminism of the sixties, when it was more of a separatist movement, but it's well beyond that now. People think you can't be a feminist and have the man pay on a date, or wear makeup or high heels. It's not about that, it's how you choose to adopt it.

—Alix, eighteen years old

Conclusion
Be True to Yourself Always

These days, I do things for myself.

I don't try to live up to some picture-perfect image. I don't dress or act in ways just to please a guy, or to come off as better than someone else. If something's on my mind, I speak up, even if it makes some waves.

—Jenna, sixteen years old

Finding our true selves—being comfortable in our own skin, thrilled with who we are, and in love with the possibilities of life—is a challenging endeavor. It's not easy to simply glide through girlhood. Amid the changes our bodies go through and the growing up we have to do, some of the ideas and images we get of ourselves and our experiences are not only hurtful but also offensive. A lot of the time we see the television hype, magazine madness, and screaming advertisements for what they are: a sham! And we know we can insist that these images and ideas echo—not drown—our own voices. We can demand that society listen up when we use our smarts and strength, form powerful connections with our peers, practice safer sex or no sex, eat what's good for us, and make great art and music. Getting in touch with ourselves can help us become even more savvy. And being able not only to ask what's wrong with the media's picture but also to say what's right with our own ideas is a big leap toward living our lives on our own terms.

Many of us are working hard to carve out some new breathing space. We are making waves and expressing ourselves through songs, protests, websites, and poetry. We are speaking out about what's important to us and going beyond the rules that hold us back. Step by step, we are developing into who we want to be—strong, comfortable, and proud. And that, my friends, is the girl power that will carry us into a rockin' womanhood. When it comes to your beauty, your body, your sexuality, and your place in this world: Enjoy and be true to yourself—always!

Notes

Note to the New Edition

1. L. J. Hofschire and B. S. Greenberg, "Media's Impact on Adolescents' Body Dissatisfaction," in *Sexual Teens, Sexual Media*, J. D. Brown et al., eds., (New Jersey: LEA Publishing, 2001).

2. D. Hargreaves, "Idealized Women in TV Ads Make Girls Feel Bad," *Journal of Social and Clinical Psychology* 21 (2002): 287–308.

3. *Teen Vogue*, June/July 2004, cover headline.

4. "Sex and Sensibility," *Washington Post Magazine*, July 16, 2000, W16.

5. Linda L. Alexander, Joan R. Cates, Nancy Herndon, and Jennifer F. Ratcliffe, eds., *Sexually Transmitted Diseases in America: How Many Cases and at What Cost?* (Menlo Park, CA: Kaiser Family Foundation, 1998): 5, 8.

Introduction

1. Wellesley College Center for Research on Women, "The AAUW Report: How Schools Shortchange Girls" (1992) (New York: Marlowe and Company, 1995).

Chapter One: The Beauty Standard

1. Ann M. Wolf, Steve L. Gortmaker, Lillian Cheung, Heather Gray, David B. Herzog, and Graham Colditz, "Activity, Inactivity, and Obesity: Racial, Ethnic, and Age Differences among Schoolgirls," *American Journal of Public Health* 83 (1993): 11.

2. Nancy C. Baker, *The Beauty Trap: Exploring Woman's Greatest Obsession* (New York: Franklin Watts, 1984).

3. Karen S. Schneider, "Mission Impossible," *People Weekly*, June 3, 1996, 64–73.

4. "Barbie Facts," Betty Bookmark, www.bettybookmark.com.

5. "Bratz Newsletter," Bratzpack, www.bratzpack.com/newsletter/newsletter.asp.

6. Susan Brownmiller, *Femininity* (New York: Linden Press/Simon and Schuster, 1984).

7. Hope Donahue, *Beautiful Stranger: A Memoir of an Obsession with Perfection* (New York: Gotham Books, 2004), 283–284.

8. Centre for Cosmetic Surgery, www.gr-cps.com (1998).

9. American Academy of Facial, Plastic, and Reconstructive Surgery, "2003 Statistics on Trends in Facial Plastic Surgery," from 2003 AAFPRS survey, www.facemd.org.

10. Harvard Eating Disorders Center, www.hedc.org.

Sidebar: Here She Comes, Miss America

1. Associated Press, "Record Low 9.8 Million Watch Miss Alabama Claim Crown," September 21, 2004. Available online at www.msn.com/id/6065619.

2. Ibid.

Sidebar: Train to be a Model

1. The Body Shop, *Full Voice* 1, 8. Available online at www.thebodyshop.com.au/infopage.cfm?topicID=49.

2. Harvard Eating Disorders Center, www.hedc.org.

Sidebar: Barbie Tales

1. "Hacking Barbie: The Barbie Liberation Organization Comes Above Ground," *Brillo*, www.brillomag.net.

2. "She's No Barbie, Nor Does She Care To Be," *The New York Times*, August 15, 1991, C11.

3. Parija Bhatnagar, "Wanna Dress Like Barbie?," money.cnn.com/2004/06/11/news/fortune500/barbie_fashion, June 14, 2004.

4. Hilary Judd and Myrica Hawker, "What Hath Barbie Wrought?," www.hardnewscafe.usu.edu/archive/nov2003.

Sidebar: Shaving, Plucking, Waxing

1. Susan A. Basow, "The Hairless Ideal: Women and Their Body Hair," *Psychology of Women Quarterly* 15 (1991): 83–96.

2. Christine Hope, "Caucasian Female Body Hair and American Culture," *Journal of American Culture* 5 (1982): 93–99.

3. Centre for Cosmetic Surgery, www.gr-cps.com, (1998).

4. Basow, 1991, 83–96.

5. Basow, 1991, 83–96

Chapter Two: Body Image

1. Alison E. Field, Lilian Cheung, Anne M. Wolf, David B. Herzog, Steven L. Gortmaker, and Graham A. Colditz, "Exposure to the Mass Media and Weight Concerns Among Girls," *Pediatrics* 103, no. 3 (March 1999), 36.

2. Nanci Hellmich, "Trying to Copy Adults Can Lead to Eating Disorders," *USA Today*, August 12, 1996, D1.

3. Jane Ogden, *Fat Chance! The Myth of Dieting Explained* (New York: Routledge, 1992), 52.

4. KA Phillips, "Body Dysmorphic Disorder: Clinical Aspects and Treatment Strategies," Bull Menninger Clin 62 (4 SupplA), (Fall 1998): A33–48.

5. Jennifer Egan, "The Thin Red Line," *The New York Times Magazine*, July 27, 1997, 20–26.

6. List drawn from the following sources: Colleen Rush, "Self-Abuse: A Cutting-Edge Addiction?" on www.drdrew.com/article.asp?id=316; and Karen Conterio and Wendy Lader, *Bodily Harm: The Breakthrough Healing Program for Self-Injurers* (New York: Hyperion, 1999).

7. Laura Shapiro, "Is Fat That Bad?" *Newsweek*, April 21, 1997, 58–64.

8. Kara Jesella, "Going Bust," *Teen Vogue*, September 2004, 204.

Sidebar: Going . . . going . . . gone?

1. E. J. Mundell, "Sitcoms, Videos Make Even Fifth-Graders Feel Fat," *Reuters Health* (Health eLine, August 26, 2002). Cited in "Media's Effect On Girls: Body Image And Gender Identity," www.mediafamily.org/facts/facts_mediaeffect.shtml.

2. J. J. Brumberg, *The Body Project: An Intimate History of American Girls* (New York: Random House, 1997), xxiv.

3. D. Hargreaves, 2002, 287–308.

4. *Mode Magazine*, June 2000.

5. White Rock Collector's Association, www.whiterocking.org.

6. A. Mazur, "U.S. Trends in Feminine Beauty and Overadaption," *Journal of Sex Research* 22 (1986): 281–303.

Sidebar: Women in Sports

1. Melpomene Institute for Women's Health, *The Bodywise Woman: Reliable Information About Physical Activity and Health* (New York: Prentice Hall Press, 1990).

2. Greta L. Cohen, *Women in Sport: Issues and Controversies* (Newbury Park, CA: Sage Publications, 1993).

Chapter Three: Eating Disorders

1. National Institute of Mental Health, *Eating Disorders* (Publication No. 94-3477), (Rockville, MD: National Institute of Mental Health, 1994).

2. Ibid.

3. C. G. Fairburn, and S.J. Beglin, "Studies of the Epidemiology of Bulimia Nervosa," *American Journal of Psychiatry* 147, no. 4 (1990): 401–408.

4. D. E. Schotte and A. J. Stunkard, "Bulimia vs. Bulimic Behaviors on a College Campus," *Journal of the American Medical Association* 258 (1987), 1213–1215.

5. P. K. Keel, J. E. Mitchell, K. B. Miller, T. L. Davis, and S. J. Crow, "Long-term Outcome of Bulimia Nervosa," *Archives of General Psychiatry* 56, no.1, 63–69.

6. National Institute of Mental Health, *Eating Disorders* (Publication No. 94-3477), (Rockville, MD: National Institute of Mental Health, 1994).

7. Leeann Alexander-Mott and D. Barry Lumsden, eds., *Understanding Eating Disorders: Anorexia Nervosa, Bulimia Nervosa, and Obesity* (Washington, D.C.: Taylor and Francis, 1994).

8. National Institute of Mental Health, *Eating Disorders* (Publication No. 94-3477), (Rockville, MD: National Institute of Mental Health, 1994).

9. Ibid.

10. Ibid.

Sidebar: Eating Disorders in History

1. Tilmann Habermas, "Friderada: A Case of Miraculous Fasting," *International Journal of Eating Disorders* 5 (1986): 555–562.

2. Linda Lewis Alexander and Judith H. LaRosa, *New Dimensions in Women's Health* (Boston: Jones and Bartlett Publishers, 1994).

Sidebar: Having an Eating Disorder

1. List drawn from the following sources: Linda Lewis Alexander and Judith H. LaRosa, *Anorexia: Dying to Be Thin* (Seattle: Life Skills Education Inc., 1996); Alexander and LaRosa, *Bulimia: Eating Yourself Sick* (Seattle: Life Skills Education Inc., 1996); Harvard Eating Disorders Center, www.hedc.org (2004).

Chapter Four: Taking a Good Look Down There

1. U.S. National Library of Medicine/Medline Plus, www.nlm.nih.gov/medlineplus.

2. Hilda Hutcherson, *What Your Mother Never Told You About S-E-X* (New York: Berkley Publishing Group, 2002), 79.

3. June M. Reinisch and Ruth Beasley, *The Kinsey Institute's New Report on Sex: What You Must Know to Be Sexually Literate* (New York: St. Martin's Press, 1990), 278.

Sidebar: Pads and Tampons . . . and Some Alternatives

1. Ada P. Kahn and Linda Hughey Holt, *The A to Z of Women's Sexuality: A Concise Encyclopedia* (Lafayette, LA: Hunter House, 1992).

2. Karen Houppert, "Pulling the Plug on the Sanitary Protection Industry," *The Village Voice*, Feb. 7, 1995.

3. The DivaCup, www.divacup.com.

Sidebar: The Hymen

1. Clellan S. Ford and Frank A. Beach, *Patterns of Sexual Behavior* (New York: Harper and Row, 1981).

Chapter Five: Coming to Terms with Our Sexuality

1. Patricia Voydanoff and Brenda W. Donnelly, *Adolescent Sexuality and Pregnancy* (Newbury Park, CA: Sage Publications, 1990).

2. Laura Stepp, "Parents are Alarmed by an Unsettling New Fad in Middle Schools: Oral Sex," *Washington Post*, July 8, 1999, A1.

3. Lisa Remez, "Oral Sex Among Adolescents: Is it Sex or is it Abstinence?" *Family Planning Perspectives* 32, no. 6 (Nov/Dec 2000): 298–304.

4. J. G. Mercer "Defining and Teaching Abstinence: An Email Survey of Health Educators," (unpublished thesis, North Carolina State University, 1999).

5. Gary Remafedi, "Sexual Orientation and Youth Suicide," *MSJAMA—Review* 282 (October 6, 1999): 1291–1292.

Sidebar: The Kinsey Scale

1. A. Kinsey, W. Pomeroy, and C. Martin, *Sexual Behavior in the Human Male* (Philadelphia: Saunders, 1948).

Sidebar: Vampire Lesbian and Other Incredible Tales

1. Joan Nestle, ed., *The Persistent Desire: A Femme-Butch Reader* (Boston: Alyson Publications, 1992), 100.

Chapter Six: Being in Charge of Our Sexuality

1. Elizabeth Terry and Jennifer Manlove, "Trends in Sexual Activity and Contraceptive Use among Teens," Washington, D.C.: National Campaign to Prevent Teen Pregnancy, 2000.

2. Jo Anne Grunbaum et al., *Youth Risk Behavior Surveillance—United States*, 2001. Morbidity & Mortality Weekly Report Surveillance Summaries 51 (SS-4), (June 28, 2002): 1–64.

3. Kaiser Family Foundation, *Communication: A Series of National Surveys of Teens about Sex*, Menlo Park, CA: Henry J. Kaiser Family Foundation, 2002.

4. Centers for Disease Control and Prevention, "National and State-Specific Pregnancy Rates among Adolescents—United States, 1995–1997," *Morbidity and Mortality Weekly Report* 49, no. 27 (July 14, 2000): 605.

5. Linda Alexander, et al. *Sexually Transmitted Diseases*, 5, 8.

6. P. J. Feldblum and J. A. Fortney, "Condoms, Spermicides, and the Transmission of Human Immunodeficiency Virus: A Review of the Literature," *American Journal of Public Health* 78 (1988), 52–54.

7. John Hutchins, *The Next Best Thing: Helping Sexually Active Teens Avoid Pregnancy*. Washington, D.C.: National Campaign to Prevent Teen Pregnancy, 2000.

8. Helene D. Gayle, *Letter to Colleagues from Helene D. Gayle, M.D., M.P.H., Director, National Center for HIV, STD, and TB Prevention*, U.S. Centers for Disease Control and Prevention, August 4, 2000.

9. H. Fu et al., "Contraceptive failure rates: New estimates from the 1995 National Survey of Family Growth," *Family Planning Perspectives* 31, no. 2 (1999): 56–63.

10. Linda J. Piccinino and William D. Mosher, "Trends in Contraceptive Use in the United States: 1982–1995," *Family Planning Perspectives* 30, no. 1 (1998): 4–10, 46.

11. Martin Vessey et al., "Mortality in Relation to Oral Contraceptive Use and Cigarette Smoking," *Lancet* 362 (July 2003): 185–191.

12. Planned Parenthood Federation of America, Inc., *Your Contraceptive Choices*, www.plannedparenthood.org/bc/cchoices2.

13. Ibid.

14. Ibid.

15. The Alan Guttmacher Institute, *Teenage Pregnancy: Overall Trends and State-by-State Information* (New York: Alan Guttmacher Institute, 1999), 5.

16. Stanley K. Henshaw, "Unintended pregnancy in the United States," *Family Planning Perspectives* 30, no. 1 (Jan/Feb 1998): 24–29, 46.

Real Girl Real World

17. The Alan Guttmacher Institute, *Teenage Pregnancy*.

18. The Alan Guttmacher Institute, *Sharing Responsibility: Women, Society and Abortion Worldwide* (New York: Alan Guttmacher Institute, 1999), chart 1.1.

19. The Alan Guttmacher Institute, *Teenage Pregnancy*.

20. Centers for Disease Control and Prevention, "Abortion Surveillance—United States, 2000." *Morbidity and Mortality Weekly Report* 52 (SS-12) (November 28, 2003).

21. Alan Guttmacher Institute, *Sex and America's Teenagers* (New York: Alan Guttmacher Institute, 1994).

22. Linda Alexander et al., *Sexually Transmitted Diseases*.

23. Hillard Weinstock, Stuart Berman, and Willard Cates, Jr., "Sexually Transmitted Diseases Among American Youth: Incidence and Prevalence Estimates, 2000," *Perspectives on Sexual and Reproductive Health* 36, no. 1 (January/February 2004): 6–10.

24. Office of Communications and Public Liaison National Institute of Allergy and Infectious Diseases, Fact Sheet (Bethesda, MD: National Institutes of Health, 1998).

25. World Health Organization, *HIV/AIDS and Adolescents: Young People—A Window of Hope in the HIV/AIDS Pandemic*, www.who.int/child-adolescent-health/HIV/HIV_adolescents.htm.

26. Advocates for Youth, *Adolescent Sexual Health in Developing Countries*, www.advocatesforyouth.org.

27. World Health Organization, *HIV/AIDS and Adolescents*.

28. Ibid.

29. Lori Heise, Mary Ellsberg, and Megan Gottemoeller, "Ending Violence Against Women," *Population Reports*, Series L, no. 11, December 1999.

30. Callie Marie Rennison and Sarah Welchans, *Bureau of Justice Special Report: Intimate Partner Violence*, May 2000.

31. The Domestic Violence Advocacy Program of Family Resources, Inc., www.acadv.org/dating.html.

Sidebar: How to Use a Condom

1. Adapted from the ASHA American Social Health Association, www.ashastd.org.

Sidebar: Which Contraceptive Methods Protect Us Against STIs?

1. Drawn from the following sources: Alexander and LaRosa, 1994; American College Health Association, *Contraception: Choosing a Method* (Baltimore: American College Health Association, 1989).

Sidebar: History of Abortion

1. Ramona I Slupik, ed., *American Medical Association's Complete Guide to Women's Health* (New York: Random House, 1996).

2. The Boston Women's Health Book Collective, *The New Our Bodies, Ourselves: A Book By and For Women* (New York: Simon and Schuster, Inc., 1992).

3. Geoffrey T. Holtz, *Welcome to the Jungle: The Why Behind "Generation X"* (New York: St. Martin's Press, 1995), 189.

Sidebar: Definitions of Sexual Assault

1. A. Parrott and L. Beckhofer, eds., *Acquaintance Rape: The Hidden Crime* (New York: Wiley Publishers, 1991).

Chapter Seven: Feminism

1. Susan J. Douglas, *Where the Girls Are: Growing Up Female with the Mass Media* (New York: New York Times Books, 1994), 278.
2. U.S. Department of Labor, Current Population Survey, Bureau of Labor Statistics 2002 annual averages.
3. The White House Project, www.thewhitehouseproject.org.
4. James T. Bond et al., *Highlights of the 2002 National Study of the Changing Work Force Data* (New York City: Families and Work Institute, 2002), 16–20.
5. Martin Reed, "Women Missing in Directing Action," *USA Today*, November 24, 2004, 2D.
6. Mara Mayor, "Fears and Fantasies of the Anti-Suffragists," *Connecticut Review* 7, no. 2 (April 1974): 64–74.
7. Ginette Castro, trans. Elizabeth Loverde-Bagwell, *American Feminism: A Contemporary History* (New York: New York University Press, 1990).
8. Douglas, *Where the Girls Are*, 146.
9. Quoted in Joseph Lelyveld, "Should Women be Nicer Than Men?" *New York Times Magazine*, April 17, 1977, 126.
10. Douglas, *Where the Girls Are*, 275.
11. Quoted in Susan Faludi, *Backlash: The Undeclared War Against American Women* (New York: Crown, 1991), 319.
12. Mayor, "Fears and Fantasies," 64–74.
13. Ibid.
14. Louise Bernikow, in association with the National Women's History Project, *The American Woman's Almanac: An Inspiring and Irreverent Women's History* (New York: Berkley Books, 1997), 3.
15. Ibid., 3.
16. Center for American Women and Politics, www.cawp.rutgers.edu.
17. Excerpts from: The Combahee River Collective Statement. Source: www.buffalostate.edu/orgs/rspms/combahee.html.
18. Quoted in Douglas, 1994, 221.
19. Center for American Women and Politics, www.cawp.rutgers.edu
20. The White House Project, www.thewhitehouseproject.org
21. Quoted in Karen Green and Tristan Taormino, eds., *A Girl's Guide to Taking Over the World: Writings from the Girl Zine Revolution* (New York: St. Martin's Griffin, 1997).

Bibliography

Note to the New Edition

Simmons, Rachel, *Odd Girl Out: The Hidden Culture of Aggression in Girls* (New York: Harcourt Brace, 2002).

Chapter 1: The Beauty Standard

Freedman, Rita Jackaway, *Beauty Bound* (Lexington, Mass.: Lexington Books, 1986).

Hansen, Joseph, Evelyn Reed, and Sonja Franeta, *Cosmetics, Fashion and the Exploitation of Woman* (New York: Pathfinder Press, 1986).

Lord, M. G., *Forever Barbie: The Unauthorized Biography of a Real Doll* (New York: William Morrow, 1994).

Ronn, Sharon, *The Changing Face of Beauty* (St. Louis: Mosby, 1992).

Stewart, Nora Kinzer, *Put Down and Ripped Off: The American Woman and the Beauty Cult* (New York: Crowell, 1977).

Wolf, Naomi, *The Beauty Myth: How Images of Beauty Are Used Against Women* (New York: William Morrow, 1991).

Chapter 2: Body Image

Blue, A., *Grace Under Pressure: The Emergence of Women in Sport* (London: Sidgwick and Jackson, 1987).

Brumberg, Joan Jacobs, *The Body Project: An Intimate History of American Girls* (New York: Random House, 1997).

Chernin, Kim, *The Obsession: Reflections on the Tyranny of Slenderness* (New York: Harper and Row, 1981).

Claiborn, James, and Cherry Pedrick, *The BDD Workbook: Overcome Body Dysmorphic Disorder and End Body Image Obsessions* (Oakland, CA: New Harbinger, 2002).

Colbin, Annemarie, *Food and Healing* (New York: Ballantine, 1996).

David, Marc, *Nourishing Wisdom: A Mind/Body Approach to Nutrition and Well-Being* (New York: Bell Tower, 1994).

Fraser, Laura, *Losing It: America's Obsession With Weight and the Industry That Feeds on It* (New York: Dutton, 1997).

Margen, Sheldon, and the editors of University of California at Berkeley Wellness Letter, *The Wellness Encyclopedia of Food and Nutrition* (New York: Rebus, 1992).

Phillips, Katharine, MD, *The Broken Mirror: Understanding and Treating Body Dysmorphic Disorder* (Oxford: Oxford University Press, 1998).

Pitchford, Paul, *Healing With Whole Foods: Asian Traditions and Modern Nutrition* (Berkeley, CA: North Atlantic Books, 2002).

Schlosser, Eric, *Fast Food Nation: The Dark Side of the All-American Meal* (New York: Perennial, 2002).

Chapter 3: Eating Disorders

American Association of University Women, *Shortchanging Girls, Shortchanging America: A Call to Action* (Washington, D.C.: American Association of University Women, 1991).

American Psychiatric Association, *Diagnostic and Statistical Manual of Mental Disorders: DSM IV* (Washington, D.C.: American Psychiatric Press, 1994).

Brumberg, Joan Jacobs, *The Body Project: An Intimate History of American Girls* (New York: Random House, 1997).

Fairburn, Christopher G., and Terence G. Wilson, eds., *Binge Eating: Nature, Assessment, and Treatment* (New York: Guilford Press, 1993).

Garner D. M., P. E. Garfinkel, W. Rochert, and M. P. Olmstead, "A Prospective Study of Eating Disorders in the Ballet," *Psychotherapy and Psychosomatics* 48 (1987), 170–5.

Gordon, Richard A., *Anorexia and Bulimia: Anatomy of a Social Epidemic* (Cambridge, Mass.: Blackwell, 1990).

Halmi, Katherine A., ed., "Eating Disorders," *Treatments of Psychiatric Disorders: A Task Force Report of the American Psychiatric Association* (Washington, D.C.: American Psychiatric Association, 1989).

Herzog, David B., "Eating Disorders," *The New Harvard Guide to Psychiatry* edited by Armand M. Nicholi, Jr. (Cambridge, Mass.: Harvard University Press, 1988).

Hsu, L. K. George, *Eating Disorders* (New York: Guilford Press, 1990).

Le Blanc, Donna, *You Can't Quit Until You Know What's Eating You: Overcoming Compulsive Eating* (Deerfield Beach, FL: Health Communications, 1990).

Lucas, Alexander R., "Eating Disorders," *Child and Adolescent Psychiatry: A Comprehensive Textbook* edited by Melvin Lewis (Baltimore: Williams and Wilkins, 1991).

Lundholm, J. K. and J. M. Littrell, "Desire for Thinness Among High School Cheerleaders: Relationships to Disordered Eating and Weight Control Behaviors," *Adolescence* 21 (1987), 573–9.

Maloney, M. J., J. McGuire, S. R. Daniels, and B. Specker, "Dieting Behavior and Eating Attitudes in Children," *Pediatrics* 84 (1989), 482–9.

Mitchell, James E., *Bulimia Nervosa* (Minneapolis: University of Minnesota Press, 1990).

Roth, Geneen, *Feeding the Hungry Heart: The Experience of Compulsive Eating* (New York: Plume, 1993).

—. *When Food is Love: Exploring the Relationship between Eating and Intimacy* (New York: Dutton, 1991).

Treasure, Janet, *Anorexia Nervosa: A Survival Guide for Families, Friends and Sufferers* (Hillsdale, N.J.: Lawrence Erlbaum Associates, Inc., 1997).

Chapter 4: Take a Good Look Down There

Alexander, Linda Lewis, and Judith H. LaRosa, *New Dimensions in Women's Health* (Boston: Jones and Bartlett Publishers, 1994).

Fausto-Sterling, Anne, *Myths of Gender: Biological Theories About Women and Men* (New York: Basic Books, 1992).

Hutcherson, Hilda, *What Your Mother Never Told You About S-E-X.* (New York: Putnam's, 2002).

Masters, W. H., V. E. Johnson, and R. C. Kologny, *Heterosexuality* (New York: HarperCollins, 1994).

Stibbs, Anne, ed., *A Woman's Place: Quotations About Women* (New York: Avon Books, 1992).

Warren, M. P., "Physical and Biological Aspects of Puberty," *Girls at Puberty: Biological and Psychosocial Perspectives* edited by J. Brook-Gunn and A. Petersen (New York: Plenum, 1983).

Chapter 5: Coming to Terms with Our Sexuality

Faderman, Lillian, ed., *Chloe Plus Olivia: An Anthology of Lesbian Literature from the Seventeenth Century to the Present* (New York: Viking, 1994).

The National Museum and Archive of Lesbian and Gay History, *The Lesbian Almanac: The Most Comprehensive Reference Source of Its Kind* (New York: Berkley Books, 1996).

Chapter 6: Being in Charge of Our Sexuality

Babikian, H. M., "Abortion," *Comprehensive Textbook of Psychiatry II* edited by A. M. Freedman, H. I. Kaplan, and B. J. Sadlock (Baltimore: Williams and Wilkins, 1975).

Herman, Judith, *Trauma and Recovery: The Aftermath of Violence—From Domestic Violence to Political Terror* (New York: Basic Books, 1992).

Masters, W. H., J. E. Johnson, and R. C. Kologny, *Heterosexuality* (New York: HarperCollins, 1994).

Mohr, J. C., *Abortion in America: The Origins and Evolution of National Policy, 1800-1900* (New York: Oxford University Press, 1978).

ORTHO Pharmaceutical Corporation, *Vaginitis: Nearly Every Woman is Affected by It: Here Are the Facts* (Raritan, N.J.: ORTHO Pharmaceutical Corp., 1994).

Chapter 7: Feminism

Abraham, Yvonne, "Third Wave Feminism: Lipstick Liberation," *The Worcester Phoenix*, May 30–June 5, 1997.

Bravo, Ellen, *The Job/Family Challenge: A 9 to 5 Guide* (New York: John Wiley and Sons, 1995).

Crocker, Elvira Valenzuela, *Mana: One Dream, Many Voices—A History of the Mexican American Women's National Association 1991*, www.hermana.org.

Davis, Marni, "Third Wave or Low Tide? The Struggles of a Young Feminist Advocacy Group," womenroom.tripod.com.

Douglas, Susan J., *Where the Girls Are: Growing Up Female with the Mass Media* (New York: New York Times Books, 1994).

Doyle, Laura, *The Surrendered Wife: A Practical Guide for Finding Intimacy, Passion, and Peace with a Man* (New York: Simon & Schuster, 2001).

Faludi, Susan, *Backlash: The Undeclared War Against American Women* (New York: Crown, 1991).

Findlen, Barbara, ed., *Listen Up: Voices from the Next Feminist Generation* (Seattle: Seal Press, 1995).

Friedan, Betty, *The Feminine Mystique* (New York: Norton, 1974).

hooks, bell, *Ain't I a Woman: Black Women and Feminism* (Boston: South End Press, 1981).

Hull, Gloria T., Patricia Bell Scott, and Barbara Smith, eds, *All the Women Are White, All the Blacks Are Men, But Some of Us Are Brave: Black Women's Studies* (Old Westbury, NY: Feminist Press, 1982).

Kramarae, Cheris, and Paula A. Treichler, *Feminist Dictionary* (Boston: Pandora Press, 1985).

Lorde, Audre, *Sister Outsider: Essays and Speeches* (Trumansburg, NY: Crossing Press, 1984).

Millett, Kate, *Sexual Politics* (Garden City, NY: Doubleday, 1970).

Paglia, Camile, *Sexual Personae: Art and Decadence from Nefertiti to Emily Dickinson* (New Haven, CT: Yale University Press, 1990).

Ryan, Mary P., *Womanhood in America: From Colonial Times to the Present* (New York: New Viewpoints, 1975).

Schlessinger, Laura, *The Proper Care and Feeding of Husbands* (New York: Harper Collins, 2004).

Sommers, Christina Hoff, *Who Stole Feminism? How Women Have Betrayed Women* (New York: Simon & Schuster, 1994).

Online Resources

The following websites were very helpful in compiling information for various sections of the book:

National Institute on Media and the Family, www.mediafamily.org

Planned Parenthood Federation of America, Inc., www.plannedparenthood.com

Harvard Eating Disorders Center, www.hedc.org

Index

empowerment: 225–228

Ensler, Eve: 221

environmental issues: 101–102

equality/equal rights, fight for: 202, 203, 208, 210, 211, 212–213

Equal Pay Act: 211

Equal Rights Amendment: 203, 212–213

Essence: 63

ethnicity: 8, 9, 10–11, 12–13, 19, 41

Evans, Jodie: 220–221

exams, breast: 108

exams, pelvic: 106–110, 166; reasons for 106; what to expect 108

exercise: 41–44, 49–54; obsession with 45

expections for sex: 123

extreme dieting: 44–45

F

fairy tales: 1, 6–7, 41

family planning clinics: 152; *see also* resources

fantasies, sexual: 114–115

fashion: 8–14; and thinness 36–41; changes in 16–20; industry 11; resources 20

fashion magazines: 3, 8–14, 21–23, 39; alternatives to 30–31, 63

fat: 54–57; liberation movement 55; resources 57

Fat!So?: 224

Faulkner, Shannon: 215

Fawcett, Farrah: 19

fear, of sexual assault: 189

Feeding the Hungry Heart: 67

feelings: 149; about sex 123–124

fellatio: 121–122

female condom: 161–162

female/male inequality: 197–199, 223–224

female sexuality: 114, 115, 119–149

FemCap: 164

Feminine Mystique, The: 211

feminism: xiv, 197–228; anti-feminists 203; as mental illness 202–203; contemporary 218–224, 225–228; definitions 198, 199; empowerment 225–228; history of 205–213; labeling of 202–203; opinions about 199–204; politics 226–227; resources 206–207, 216, 222–223, 224–225, 226–227

feminist organizations: 211, 213; for women of color 211, 216–217

Ferraro, Geraldine: 215

"first-time" stories: 125–127

fitness: 49–54; regimens 44–45; tips 50–51

flappers: 18

Flashdance: 19

"flaws," obsession with: 45–46

food: books about 69; obsession with 68, 71–72; *see also* eating disorders

foreplay: 122

Franklin, Aretha: 19

Freud, Sigmund: 114, 142

Friedan, Betty: 199, 210

Friends: 23, 37

friends, helping: 82–84

"friends with benefits": 120

Fulcher, Sarah: 53

F-word: 204

G

G.I. Joes: 15, 16

Garbo, Greta: 18

Gardner, Ava: 18

gays: and HIV/AIDS 186; bashing 141; rights 146–148

genital herpes: 183

genital warts: 184

Gibson Girl: 17

Ginsburg, Ruth Bader: 214

girdles: 18–19

girl power: 229–230

Girl's Guide to Taking Over the World: Writings from the Girl Zine Revolution: 224

girls, prettiness of: 1

"giving head": 121–122

Glamour: 13, 63

"going down": 121–122

Gompers, Samuel: 5

gonorrhea (dose, drip, clap): 183, 184

Gorman, Margaret: 5

Green, Karen: 224

Grrrls: 198, 219

grunge: 19

G-spot (Grafenberg spot): 113–114

Guerrilla Girls: 219–220; writings by 220

Gyn/Ecology: The Metaethics of Radical Feminism: 211–212

gynecologists: 106–110

H

hair: 23–26; feathered 19; shaving of 25

Hamm, Mia: 53

Hanna, Kathleen: 219

harassment: 191; *see also* sexual assault

hatred: of men 199, 202, 204, 211; of women 198

Hayworth, Rita: 18

health: and eating disorders 86–87; books about 109; issues 116–117; organizations 116–117

healthy eating: 49–51, resources 51, 53–54

help, with eating disorders: 82–85

hepatitis-B (serum hepatitis): 183–184

herpes: 183

hippies: 19

history: of abortion 178–179; of feminism 205–213

HIV/AIDS: 185–186; and condoms 153; *see also* acquired immune deficiency syndrome

homophobia: 140–145

homosexuality: 134–149; *see also* lesbianism/bisexuality

"hooking up": 120

hooks, bell, writings by: 217

hormones: 166–167; sex hormones 97, 99

hotlines: for eating disorders 84; emergency contraception 182; gays/lesbians 141, 146, 147; HIV/AIDS 186; safer sex 159; self-injury 47; sexual assault 190; sexually transmitted infections (STIs) 189

household chores: 198

housewives: 18, 210

HPV (human papillomavirus): 184

Hull, Gloria T.: 212

Acknowledgments

We are thrilled to have the opportunity to update *Real Girl Real World* and to offer so many pages of new resources, information, and interviews with girls. It has been ten years and a long journey since we first sat down together and said, "Let's write a book. . . ." We could never have brought this dream into reality without the support of many individuals.

Our first thanks are to the wonderful staff (and former staff) at Seal Press and Avalon Publishing Group. Thank you for believing in this book and putting your faith in us. We feel so fortunate to have found a publisher who shares our passion for creating a book that we wish we could have read as girls. Thank you to the first group of editors who helped with our first edition. Thank you to our current editors, Ingrid Emerick and Mansa Solís, whose thoughtful comments make our writing shine. Thank you to Denise Silva and Maggie Friedland for all of their assistance in gathering the latest facts and resources. Thanks also to Ellen Forney for her unique and wonderful illustrations.

Special thanks from Samantha goes to: Bruno de Oliveira, for his love and encouragement to always "subir a montanha." And a toast to my friends: Mia (for always making me laugh even with Laura banging on the laptop), Silvia and Catherine (for your thoughts in the Algarve), Andrea, Diana, and Lucianna (for being the coolest moms in Miami), Gio and Zisca (for your friendship and knowledge), Tirene (for cuddling Laura the perfect way), and Mary Jane (for your writing encouragement). And to all my family for their loving support, especially Michael and Heather for their grounding voices, and Sissy—for caring and for being "family" too. And thank you to my daughters, Sophia (six) and Laura (almost one), for your joyous and delightful spirits. I am very thankful to my father, Lewis Phillips, in loving memory, for his kind nature and for always citing those literary references.

And special thanks from Heather goes to: Dad, Angie, and my sisters (Anne, Dawn, and Susan) for your loving support and enthusiasm for my many projects, including *Real Girl Real World*. And to Susan, my twin, who is always there to offer writing encouragement and willing to be my dream weaver. Thank you to my special writing group, the ladies, Claire, Liza, Robin, and Sally—whose friendships mean so much and who are always inspiring me. Thank you also to Irene, who rubbed my feet; Shay, who sat on the beach and discussed our futures; Elle B, who feng shui'd and wrote superstar songs; Brooke, who put it all in an energy vortex for me; and Gilly, for her beautiful poem and friendship. Thank you to Charlie for hugs, love, and support. And finally I'd like to send some love to my nieces (Devon, Lauren, and Lily) and nephews (Jay, Conner, and Gage) who brighten up my life.

For their expert opinions, we'd also like to thank Sigi Weiss, Barrie Dolnick, David Herzog, MD, director of the Harvard Eating Disorders Center at Massachusetts General Hospital, and Marcy Bloom at Aradia Women's Health Center.

Finally, and most importantly, we thank all the girls we interviewed: This book would not exist without you. We are keeping your identities anonymous, but we remember each and every one of you with clarity. You were our partners, and we are grateful for the hours you spent with us, sharing your souls and helping us create a different, bolder vision for girls.

Credits

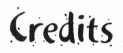

About the Authors

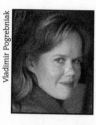

HEATHER GRAY grew up with three sisters and so has been dealing with girl issues for a lifetime. She graduated with a bachelor's degree in psychology from Brown University in 1990 and landed her first job as a research assistant for the Harvard Eating Disorder Center's long-term study of girls and women with eating disorders. This experience led to her interest in inspiring girls to empower themselves rather than listening to the mixed-up messages we receive from so many sources. After getting her master's degree in public health from the University of North Carolina, she moved to New York City to write *Real Girl Real World* with Samantha Phillips. Heather currently lives in the West Village of New York City, where she continues to create inspiration through writing, Reiki, nutritional counseling, and public health consulting.

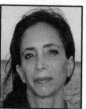

SAMANTHA PHILLIPS graduated with a bachelor's degree in comparative literature from Brown University in 1990 and received a master's degree in education from Lesley College. She is currently a freelance writer for numerous magazines and newspapers and a contributing writer for *Fit Pregnancy* magazine. She is a part-time lecturer at the University of Miami, where she has taught freshman writing classes. She lives in Miami with her husband, Bruno, and daughters, Sophia and Laura. Under duress, she did give Sophia a Barbie when she turned three (aah) and her family now has a tangled collection of disheveled Barbies that live mostly in a drawer. She is presently working on a new project with Heather.

About the Illustrator

ELLEN FORNEY's work has appeared in many publications including *LA Weekly*, *The Stranger*, *BUST*, *Nickelodeon*, and *The Stranger*. Her book of autobiographical comic strips, *Monkey Food: The Complete "I Was Seven in '75" Collection* (Fantagraphics Books), was nominated for several national comics awards. She has been teaching courses on comics at Cornish College of the Arts since 2002. More of her work is at www.ellenforney.com.

Selected Titles from Seal Press

For more than 25 years, Seal Press has published groundbreaking books. By women. For women. Visit our website at www.sealpress.com.

Listen Up: Voices from the Next Feminist Generation edited by Barbara Findlen. $16.95, 1-58005-054-9. A revised and expanded edition of the Seal Press classic, this anthology features the voices of a new generation of women expressing the vibrancy and vitality of today's feminist movement.

Colonize This!: Young Women of Color on Today's Feminism edited by Daisy Hernández and Bushra Rehman. $16.95, 1-58005-067-0. This diverse collection of some of today's brightest new voices takes on identity, family, class, and the notion that feminism is one cohesive movement.

The F-Word: Feminism in Jeopardy by Kristin Rowe-Finkbeiner. $14.95, 1-58005-114-6. An astonishing look at the tenuous state of women's rights and issues in America, this pivotal book also incites women with voting power to change their situations.

Cunt: A Declaration of Independence by Inga Muscio. $14.95, 1-58005-075-1. An ancient title of respect for women, "cunt" long ago veered off the path of honor and now careens toward the heart of every woman as an expletive. Muscio traces this winding road, giving women both the motivation and the tools to claim "cunt" as a positive and powerful force in the lives of all women.

Cinderella's Big Score: Women of the Punk and Indie Underground by Maria Raha. $15.95, 1-58005-116-2. Women not only rock as hard as the boys, but they also test the limits of what is culturally acceptable in this tribute to the women of punk rock.

Secrets and Confidences: The Complicated Truth about Women's Friendships edited by Karen Eng. $14.95, 1-58005-112-X. This frank, funny, and poignant collection acknowledges the complex relationships between girlfriends.